Total Joint Arthroplasty - Challenges, Advances and Clinical Insights

Edited by Alessandro Rozim Zorzi

Published in London, United Kingdom

Total Joint Arthroplasty - Challenges, Advances and Clinical Insights
http://dx.doi.org/10.5772/intechopen.1005940
Edited by Alessandro Rozim Zorzi

Contributors
Abdul Sathar, Ahmed Aly Naggar, Alaa Aldeen Eydou, Alessandro Rozim Zorzi, Arthur Luiz Correia de Medeiros, Deepak Jain, Devang Bharti, Glenda Feldberg, Gustavo Enrique Barros, Harpal Singh Selhi, James M. Broderick, James Toale, Janaina Bosso Ricciardi, Khalid Al Hamadi, Mohamed Ahmed, Mohamed Ragab, Muhammad Thahir, Rajnish Garg, Ravindra Mohan, Rodrigo Hamada, Roshan Pais, Shaher Hasanain, Sumit Anand, Tushar Jethi, Varun Narula

First published in London, United Kingdom, 2025 by IntechOpen
IntechOpen is the global imprint of INTECHOPEN LIMITED, registered in England and Wales, registration number: 11086078, 167-169 Great Portland Street, London, W1W 5PF, United Kingdom

For EU product safety concerns: IN TECH d.o.o., Prolaz Marije Krucifikse Kozulić 3, 51000 Rijeka, Croatia, info@intechopen.com or visit our website at intechopen.com.

British Library Cataloguing-in-Publication Data
A catalogue record for this book is available from the British Library

Total Joint Arthroplasty - Challenges, Advances and Clinical Insights
Edited by Alessandro Rozim Zorzi
p. cm.
Print ISBN 978-1-83635-097-2
Online ISBN 978-1-83635-096-5
eBook (PDF) ISBN 978-1-83635-098-9

Meet the editor

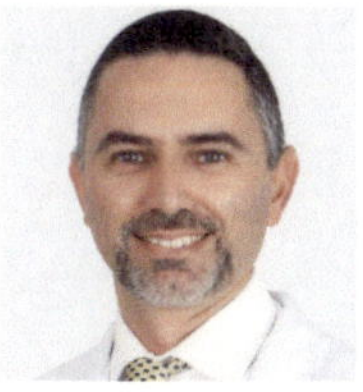

Alessandro Rozim Zorzi is a Professor of Undergraduate and Graduate Programs in Medical Sciences at São Leopoldo Mandic Medical School and a researcher in the fields of Knee Surgery and Cartilage Cell Therapy. He is a member of the Knee Surgery Medical Care Group at Hospital Israelita Albert Einstein and serves on the Regenerative Medicine Committee of the Brazilian Society of Orthopedics and Traumatology (SBOT). He serves as an orthopedic surgeon at the Clinics Hospital of the University of Campinas (UNICAMP). Dr. Zorzi earned his medical degree from the Ribeirão Preto Medical School of the University of São Paulo (USP) in 1999 and holds a Master's and Ph.D. in Surgical Sciences from UNICAMP, with additional specialization in Clinical Research from Harvard Medical School and in Research Ethics involving Human Subjects from UNESCO.

Contents

Preface

This edited volume brings together diverse perspectives on the evolving field of joint arthroplasty, with a particular focus on total knee and hip replacement. The book was developed to provide orthopedic surgeons, researchers, and allied health professionals with a comprehensive and practical overview of contemporary issues, techniques, and innovations in joint reconstruction surgery.

The chapters included in this volume reflect the collaborative work of international experts who share clinical experience, critical analysis, and evidence-based practices related to joint replacement. Topics covered span from surgical planning and implant alignment to complication management, postoperative rehabilitation, and considerations for complex or revision cases. The content aims to support decision-making in everyday practice while also offering valuable insights for academic research and future developments in the field.

Rather than promoting a single approach or philosophy, this book emphasizes the importance of individualized care, multidisciplinary collaboration, and ongoing refinement of surgical techniques based on patient needs and evolving evidence. It is intended to serve as both a reference and a stimulus for reflection and innovation among professionals dedicated to improving outcomes in joint arthroplasty.

We are grateful to all contributing authors for their expertise and commitment to advancing orthopedic knowledge. We also extend our appreciation to the editorial and production teams at IntechOpen for their support throughout the publication process.

Special thanks to the assistants and peer reviewers whose contributions were essential to the completion of this volume.

Alessandro Rozim Zorzi
Faculdade São Leopoldo Mandic,
Campinas-SP, Brazil

Chapter 1

Total Knee Arthroplasty in People with Hemophilia

Alessandro Rozim Zorzi, Arthur Luiz Correia de Medeiros, Glenda Feldberg and Janaina Bosso Ricciardi

Abstract

Hemophilic arthropathy is a severe, progressive joint disease resulting from recurrent bleeding episodes, predominantly affecting the knee joint due to its biomechanical demands. Chronic hemarthrosis leads to synovitis, cartilage degeneration, deformities, and functional impairment, severely impacting patient quality of life. Total knee arthroplasty (TKA) represents the definitive treatment in advanced stages, significantly reducing pain and restoring mobility. However, surgical management of hemophilic patients poses unique challenges, including meticulous perioperative hemostatic control, higher infection risks, and the necessity for individualized implant selection due to frequent joint deformities and compromised ligament integrity. Preoperative evaluation requires detailed clinical and radiographic assessment, emphasizing mechanical axis alignment and joint stability to determine implant type and degree of constraint. Surgical approaches must ensure comprehensive synovectomy and adequate joint exposure, minimizing persistent postoperative synovitis and bleeding. Postoperative management includes rigorous hematologic surveillance, multimodal analgesia, targeted rehabilitation, and vigilant infection prevention strategies. This chapter discusses evidence-based approaches and practical recommendations for successfully performing TKA in hemophilia patients, highlighting contemporary surgical techniques, perioperative protocols, potential complications, and emerging advances, aiming to enhance patient outcomes and facilitate clinical decision-making in this complex patient population.

Keywords: hemophilia, arthropathy, total knee arthroplasty, joint replacement, perioperative management

1. Introduction

Hemophilic arthropathy is a progressive, chronic joint disease resulting from repeated intra-articular hemorrhages, predominantly affecting individuals with hemophilia (PWH). Ankle, knee, and elbow are the most frequent sites of joint disease. The knee is particularly vulnerable due to its large size, substantial load-bearing responsibility, and frequent involvement in physical activities [1, 2].

Recurrent joint bleeds trigger chronic inflammation, causing synovial hypertrophy, cartilage degeneration, and eventual joint deterioration. Over time, this leads to severe morbidity, impaired mobility, chronic pain, and diminished quality of life. Hemophilia, an X-linked recessive disorder, affects approximately 1 in 10,000 males globally, emphasizing the importance of comprehensive clinical management strategies [3].

Patients with hemophilic knee arthropathy typically present with symptoms such as recurrent swelling, chronic pain, joint stiffness, and significant limitation in range of motion. Early on, symptoms coincide with acute episodes of hemarthrosis and may be intermittent. With disease progression, however, patients experience persistent discomfort, tenderness along the joint line, crepitus, and development of fixed flexion deformities. Physical examination often reveals joint effusion and substantial impairment in weight-bearing capabilities [4].

Accurate differential diagnosis is crucial, as symptoms overlap with conditions like osteoarthritis, rheumatoid arthritis, septic arthritis, and pigmented villonodular synovitis. Clinical evaluations, thorough patient history, laboratory assessments of coagulation factors, and advanced imaging techniques such as MRI and ultrasonography are indispensable for proper diagnosis and staging [5, 6].

The Arnold-Hilgartner radiographic classification system (**Table 1**), widely employed in clinical practice, categorizes hemophilic arthropathy into stages based on severity, guiding appropriate therapeutic interventions. This system ranges from early synovitis with minimal joint alterations to advanced disease stages characterized by extensive cartilage erosion, subchondral cyst formation, osteophytes, and eventual ankylosis [7].

2. Indications for total knee arthroplasty (TKA)

When conservative approaches—such as prophylactic factor replacement, physiotherapy, and synovectomy—fail to manage symptoms adequately, surgical interventions are indicated. Surgical candidacy is generally based on persistent joint bleeding despite optimal medical management, severe chronic pain affecting daily activities, substantial functional limitations, and advanced joint deterioration (Arnold-Hilgartner 4 or 5). Alternative surgical treatments, including arthroscopic or open synovectomy and corrective osteotomy, might be beneficial in earlier stages or younger patients. Nevertheless, TKA remains the definitive solution for severe cases of hemophilic knee arthropathy, despite the complexities posed by the underlying bleeding disorder (**Figure 1**) [8–12].

Stage	Description	Radiographic findings
0	Normal	No evidence of joint disease
1	Pre-radiographic	Soft tissue swelling, no bone changes
2	Early	Osteopenia, epiphyseal overgrowth, no joint space narrowing
3	Moderate	Joint space narrowing, subchondral cysts, osteophytes
4	Advanced	Severe joint space narrowing, bone erosions
5	End Stage	Joint destruction, fibrous or bony ankylosis, gross deformities

Table 1.
Arnold-Hilgartner radiographic classification system for staging hemophilic arthropathy.

DOI: http://dx.doi.org/10.5772/intechopen.1010667

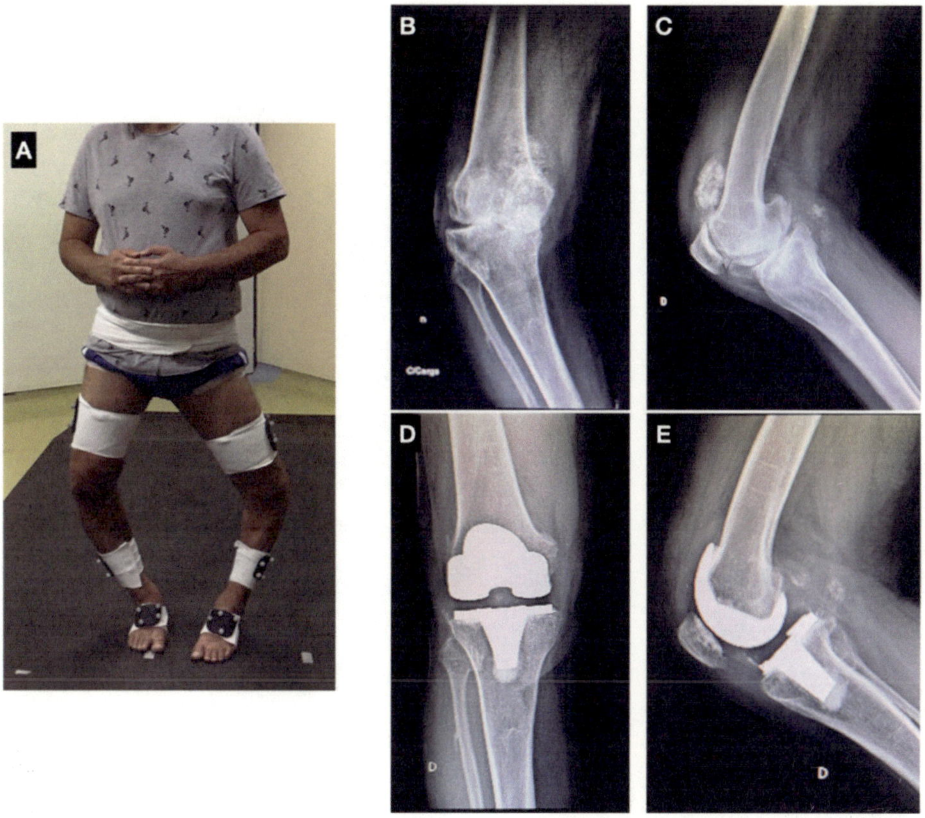

Figure 1.
(A) Clinical photograph demonstrating significant bilateral knee deformities in a patient with hemophilia, presenting severe refractory pain, functional limitation with impaired ambulation, and difficulty changing position, substantially impacting quality of life. (B) Preoperative anteroposterior knee radiograph illustrating advanced hemophilic arthropathy classified as Arnold-Hilgartner stage 4. (C) Preoperative lateral knee radiograph highlighting extensive joint damage and synovial chondromatosis. (D) Postoperative anteroposterior radiograph showing total knee arthroplasty implant in situ*, with restored joint alignment. (E) Postoperative lateral radiograph demonstrating correct prosthesis positioning and alignment.*

3. Preoperative management

Optimal outcomes in hemophilic patients undergoing TKA require meticulous perioperative planning. Achieving precise hemostatic control through individualized administration of clotting factor concentrates—guided by current international consensus and protocols, including guidelines provided by the World Federation of Hemophilia—is essential. Patients with factor VIII or IX inhibitors require specialized management using bypassing agents or newer non-factor therapies, substantially increasing perioperative complexity.

Collaboration among multidisciplinary teams involving hematologists, orthopedic surgeons, anesthesiologists, and physiotherapists is critical to minimize bleeding risks, reduce perioperative complications, and ensure successful surgical outcomes. Preoperative assessments should also address potential co-morbidities, nutritional status, and infection risks.

Prosthesis planning involves a thorough clinical evaluation of the knee to assess the range of motion, existing deformities and their reducibility, as well as the stability

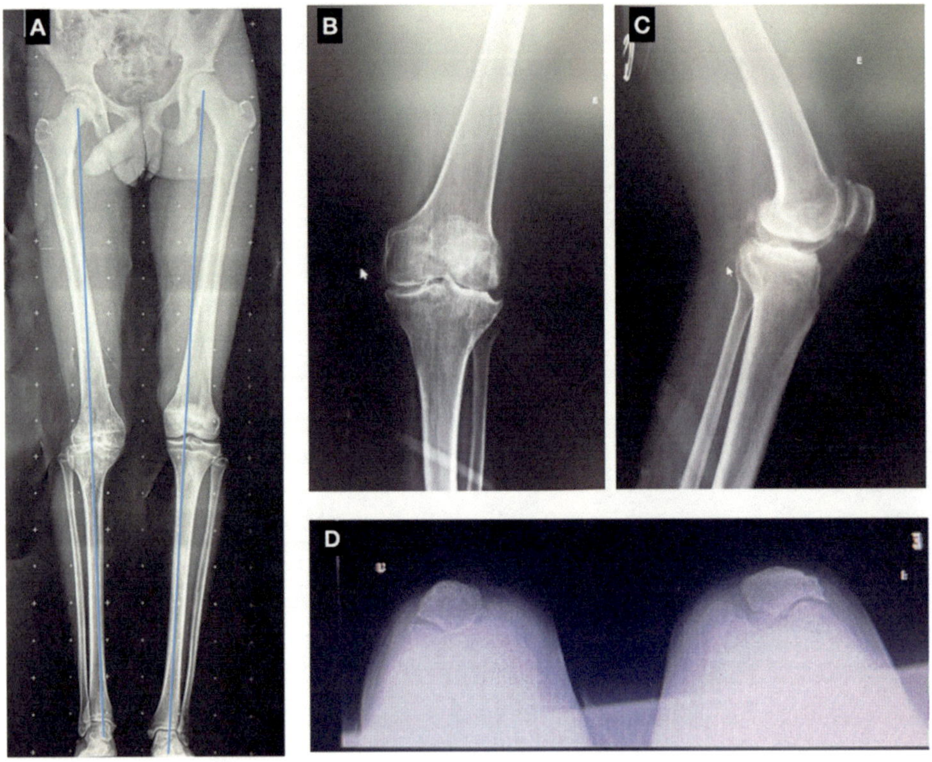

Figure 2.
Basic radiographic studies required for surgical planning in patients with hemophilic knee arthropathy. (A) Panoramic standing radiograph of the lower limbs demonstrating mechanical axes drawn from the center of the femoral head to the center of the talus. (B) Weight-bearing anteroposterior radiograph of the knee. (C) Lateral radiograph of the knee used to evaluate tibial slope and patellar height, illustrating the classic "squared patella" sign characteristic of hemophilic arthropathy. (D) Axial patellar radiograph for detailed evaluation of patellofemoral alignment and joint integrity.

of the collateral ligaments. These factors guide the selection of the appropriate degree of implant constraint during surgery. Weight-bearing radiographs are essential components of the preoperative evaluation. A standing panoramic lower limb radiograph is critical for determining the mechanical axis alignment. Knee radiographs should include at least three views: monopodal weight-bearing anteroposterior, lateral view with 30 degrees of knee flexion, and patellar axial view (**Figure 2**). Depending on the clinical findings, additional stress radiographs under varus and valgus load conditions may be necessary to complement the patient's preoperative assessment.

4. Surgical technique

Standard intraoperative practices include the administration of prophylactic antibiotics, rigorous clotting factor management, and intravenous tranexamic acid to minimize bleeding. Typically, a medial parapatellar approach provides optimal exposure, though extended surgical techniques such as quadriceps snip or tibial tubercle osteotomy might be required for ankylosed or severely deformed knees. In fixed valgus deformities, Keblish's lateral parapatellar approach is recommended.

An important difference is the excessive synovitis and widespread adhesions, characteristic findings in hemophilic knees, which necessitate meticulous release and complete synovectomy prior to prosthetic implantation (**Figure 3**).

Accurate identification and reconstruction of the joint line, frequently distorted due to severe deformities like patella baja, are pivotal to restoring appropriate knee mechanics. Surgeons rely on anatomical landmarks such as epicondyles and tibial tuberosity to guide accurate bone resections. Complex cases with severe bone loss

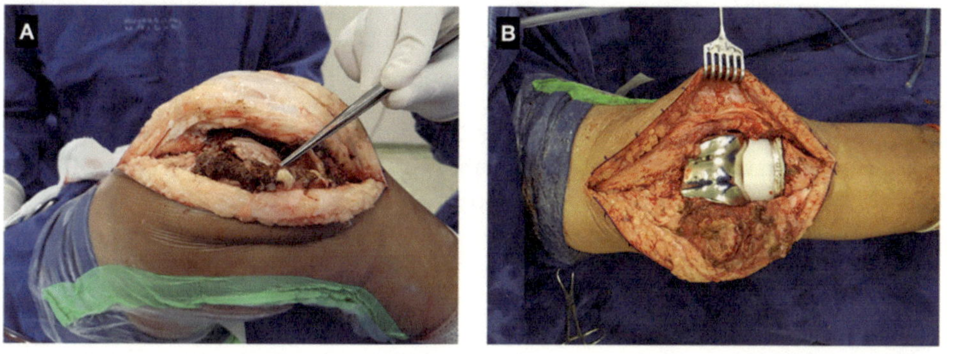

Figure 3.
(A) Intraoperative photograph showing a medial parapatellar approach, highlighting difficulty in luxating the patella due to extensive adhesions and abundant brownish synovial tissue caused by hemosiderin deposition. (B) Post-implantation photograph demonstrating the prosthesis in place and the joint cavity cleared of pathological synovial tissue following an extensive synovectomy. Minimally invasive surgical approaches are not recommended in these cases; the chosen approach must provide good exposure to ensure complete removal of inflamed synovium, thus preventing persistent synovitis, postoperative pain, and joint effusion.

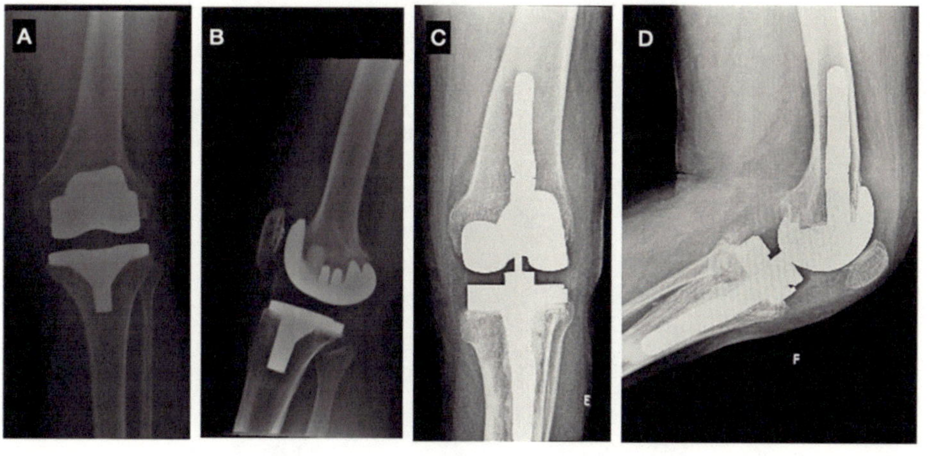

Figure 4.
Implant selection in hemophilic knee arthropathy is influenced by multiple factors, including patient age and the extent of bone deformity. Many patients are relatively young, often in their third or fourth decade of life, making preservation of bone stock crucial. Therefore, implants that do not require box preparation in the distal femur are preferred. (A-B) Anteroposterior and lateral radiographs of a primary cemented total knee arthroplasty with ultra-congruent polyethylene inserts. Cruciate-retaining implants are generally avoided due to compromised cruciate ligaments and significant joint deformities. Note the mismatch between the standard femoral component diameter and the widened femoral metaphysis commonly seen in hemophilic patients; customized implants may be required in some cases. (C-D) Anteroposterior and lateral radiographs demonstrating a semi-constrained implant with stems and augmentation blocks indicated for correction of severe joint deformities and substantial ligamentous instability.

or deformities may require advanced techniques like intraoperative fluoroscopy, navigation-assisted surgery, and augmentation strategies with stemmed prostheses to ensure proper alignment and stability (**Figure 4**).

Soft tissue and ligament balancing in hemophilic knees can be particularly challenging due to long-standing deformities and contractures. Comprehensive soft tissue releases and posterior capsular release often become necessary. Semi-constrained or constrained prosthetic implants are frequently utilized to achieve joint stability, especially when ligament integrity is compromised. Patellar management decisions—including resurfacing, realignment, or retention—should be individualized based on specific patellar pathology and tracking patterns [13, 14].

Achieving meticulous hemostasis throughout the procedure is essential. Strategies including pneumatic tourniquet use, topical tranexamic acid application, and precise vessel cauterization significantly reduce postoperative bleeding complications. Cement fixation of implants, preferably antibiotic-loaded, is recommended to enhance fixation quality in typically osteopenic hemophilic bone.

5. Postoperative care

Postoperative care focuses on vigilant monitoring and management of factor levels to minimize bleeding risk, alongside careful infection control measures due

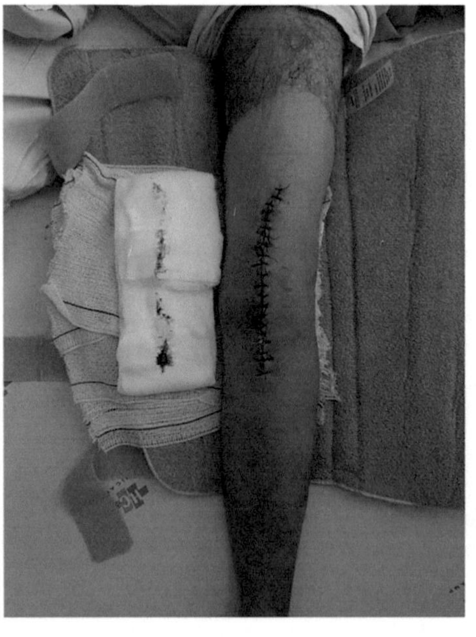

Figure 5.
First postoperative day. The initial wound dressing must be opened in the presence of both the orthopedic surgeon and the hematologist to accurately evaluate postoperative bleeding by inspecting gauze dressings and any blood discharge from the surgical incision. This assessment guides appropriate adjustments in clotting factor dosage during the immediate postoperative period. Tranexamic acid is maintained for the first five postoperative days. Early mobilization, including ambulation with a walker, is encouraged from the first postoperative day if pain and bleeding are adequately controlled. In cases of significant bleeding, temporary rest is recommended. Multimodal analgesia and ultrasound-guided adductor canal nerve blocks significantly enhance patient comfort and facilitate rehabilitation in the initial postoperative days.

Phases	Description	Objectives
1	Postoperative (Week 1–4)	Control pain and swelling, improve range of motion (0–90 degrees), achieve full extension, and begin weight-bearing as tolerated. CPM device is indicated if previous joint stiffness.
2	Early recovery (Week 4–8)	Increase range of motion (90–120 degrees), improve quadriceps and hamstring strength, normalize gait pattern, and reduce reliance on assistive devices. Hydrotherapy is a valuable resource following suture removal and wound healing.
3	Mid-recovery (Week 8–12)	Achieve full range of motion, improve muscle strength and endurance, enhance functional mobility (stairs, squatting), and return to low-impact activities.
4	Late recovery (Week 12–24)	Restore normal muscle strength and function, improve proprioception and balance, and return to pre-injury activity levels.
5	Maintenance (Beyond 24 weeks)	Maintain strength, flexibility, and function, prevent re-injury, and engage in regular exercise and activity.

Table 2.
The stages of physiotherapy rehabilitation for PWH who have undergone knee replacement surgery.

to impaired wound healing potential (**Figure 5**). Prophylactic antibiotics and strict aseptic protocols are critical components of postoperative management.

Thromboembolic prophylaxis remains controversial due to balancing bleeding risks and thrombotic potential, necessitating individualized assessment and monitoring [15].

Rehabilitation aims for gradual mobilization and structured physiotherapy to restore range of motion, strength, and functional capacity, with guidance from therapists specialized in hemophilia management. Continuous passive motion (CPM) devices may aid early postoperative recovery but should be employed cautiously to avoid bleeding complications (**Table 2**).

6. Conclusion

Managing hemophilic knee arthropathy with total knee arthroplasty demands a thorough, multidisciplinary approach involving careful perioperative planning, precise hemostatic management, meticulous surgical technique, and comprehensive rehabilitation. Ongoing advancements in hemophilia treatments, including extended half-life clotting factors, gene therapy, and novel orthopedic implants, promise significant improvements in surgical outcomes and quality of life. Continued international cooperation, education, and resource allocation are vital to expanding access to high-quality hemophilia care, especially in regions with limited resources.

Author details

Alessandro Rozim Zorzi[1,2]*, Arthur Luiz Correia de Medeiros[2], Glenda Feldberg[1] and Janaina Bosso Ricciardi[1]

1 Hemocentro UNICAMP, Department of Internal Medicine, School of Medical Sciences, University of Campinas, Campinas, SP, Brazil

2 Faculdade Sao Leopoldo Mandic, Campinas, SP, Brazil

*Address all correspondence to: arzorzi@hc.unicamp.br

References

[1] Gualtierotti R, Solimeno LP, Peyvandi F. Hemophilic arthropathy: Current knowledge and future perspectives. Journal of Thrombosis and Haemostasis. 2021;**19**(9):2112-2121. DOI: 10.1111/jth.15444 Epub 2021 Jul 27

[2] Luck JV Jr, Silva M, Rodriguez-Merchan EC, Ghalambor N, Zahiri CA, Finn RS. Hemophilic arthropathy. The Journal of the American Academy of Orthopaedic Surgeons. 2004;**12**(4):234-245. DOI: 10.5435/00124635-200407000-00004

[3] Mehta P, AKR R. Hemophilia. 2023. In: StatPearls. Treasure Island (FL): StatPearls Publishing. p. 2025

[4] Kizilocak H, Young G. Diagnosis and treatment of hemophilia. Clinical Advances in Hematology and Oncology. 2019;**17**(6):344-351

[5] Tiede A, Collins P, Knoebl P, Teitel J, Kessler C, Shima M, et al. International recommendations on the diagnosis and treatment of acquired hemophilia a. Haematologica. 2020;**105**(7):1791-1801. DOI: 10.3324/haematol.2019.230771. Epub 2020 May 7

[6] Dunn AL. Pathophysiology, diagnosis and prevention of arthropathy in patients with haemophilia. Haemophilia. 2011;**17**(4):571-578. DOI: 10.1111/j.1365-2516.2010.02472.x. Epub 2011 Feb 22

[7] Arnold WD, Hilgartner MW. Hemophilic arthropathy. Current concepts of pathogenesis and management. The Journal of Bone and Joint Surgery. American Volume. 1977;**59**(3):287-305

[8] Ingerslev J, Hvid I, Surgery in hemophilia. The general view: Patient selection, timing, and preoperative assessment. Seminars in Hematology. 2006;**43**(Suppl. 1):S23-S26. DOI: 10.1053/j.seminhematol.2005.11.024

[9] Beckers G, Massé V, Barry J, St-Louis J, Isler M, Vendittoli PA, et al. Clinical outcomes of total knee arthroplasty in patients who have hemophilic arthropathy: A prospective study. The Journal of Arthroplasty. 2024;**S0883-5403**(24):00722-00728. DOI: 10.1016/j.arth.2024.07.020 Epub ahead of print

[10] Beckers G, Massé V, Vendittoli PA, Morcos MW. Primary total knee arthroplasty in hemophilic arthropathy. EFORT Open Rev. 2023;**8**(11):830-840. DOI: 10.1530/EOR-23-0101

[11] Moore MF, Tobase P, Allen DD. Meta-analysis: Outcomes of total knee arthroplasty in the haemophilia population. Haemophilia. 2016;**22**(4):e275-e285. DOI: 10.1111/hae.12885

[12] Rodriguez-Merchan EC. Total knee replacement in haemophilic arthropathy. Journal of Bone and Joint Surgery. British Volume (London). 2007;**89**(2):186-188. DOI: 10.1302/0301-620X.89B2.18682

[13] Vahabi A, Kaya Biçer E, Aydoğdu S. Total knee arthroplasty in hemophilic knees requires its own learning phase: Lessons learned from 90 cases. The Knee. 2025;**53**:28-34. DOI: 10.1016/j.knee.2024.11.024 Epub 2024 Dec 12

[14] Mortazavi SJ, Bagheri N, Farhoud A, Hadi Kalantar S, Ghadimi E. Total knee arthroplasty in patients with hemophilia: What do we know? 2020;**8**(4):470-478. DOI: 10.22038/abjs.2019.42247.2149

[15] Zhang Q, Zhao L, Riva N, Yu Z, Jiang M, Gatt A, et al. Incidence of deep venous thrombosis in patients with hemophilia undergoing bilateral simultaneous total knee arthroplasty: A retrospective cohort study. BMC Musculoskeletal Disorders. 2024;**25**(1):326. DOI: 10.1186/s12891-024-07404-2

Chapter 2

Rotational Alignment of Tibial Component in Total Knee Arthroplasty

Muhammad Thahir, Ahmed Aly Naggar, Shaher Hasanain, Mohamed Ragab, Alaa Aldeen Eydou, Abdul Sathar, Roshan Pais and Khalid Al Hamadi

Abstract

Despite the success of TKA, rotational alignment remains an unresolved issue. The rotational alignment of the femoral component in total knee arthroplasty is generally well understood. In contrast, there is considerable debate regarding the ideal rotational alignment for the tibial component. There are well-established femoral rotational reference axes, which include: the trans-epicondylar axis (TEA), the posterior condylar axis (PCA), the whiteside line grand piano sign. All are solid and reliable references. However, in tibia, TEA could not be projected on the tibia plateau. The rotational alignment of tibial prosthesis in total knee replacement is crucial for optimal knee biomechanics, patellofemoral tracking, and long-term prosthesis survival. Component malrotation in total knee arthroplasty has been associated with poor outcomes after TKA, including persistent pain, stiffness, and patellofemoral complications. Hence, assessing rotational alignment during total knee replacement surgery plays a vital role in the outcome of the surgery. Different landmarks have been reported in the literature to guide rotational alignment of the tibia during tibial prosthesis preparation, including static and dynamic landmarks.

Keywords: total knee replacement, rotational alignment, tibial landmarks, kinematic techniques, tibial components malrotation, tibial rotation measurement, tibial malrotation complications

1. Introduction

Total knee replacement (TKR) is considered a highly effective and cost-efficient approach for alleviating pain and enhancing functionality in patients with advanced knee osteoarthritis, especially when conservative treatments fail. The procedure provides a high success rate, a low incidence of complications, and an increasing projected longevity of the implants. Nevertheless, research indicates that up to 20% of patients may still express dissatisfaction after undergoing TKR [1, 2].

A successful outcome in TKR depends on multiple factors. Patient factors, implant characteristics, and surgical technique, which appear to play important roles in achieving acceptable results. However, some patients experience poor outcomes even though physical examination and plain radiographs fail to identify any specific problem. In these cases, increased emphasis has been placed on the assessment of the rotational alignment of the femoral and tibial components [3].

Component malrotation in total knee arthroplasty has been associated with poor outcomes after TKA, including persistent pain, stiffness, and patellofemoral complications, which increase the risk of revision surgery and poor outcome [4–6].

The trans epicondylar axis and the antero-posterior axis (Whiteside's Line) of the distal femur are considered widely accepted and reliable landmarks to determine the rotational alignment of the femoral component. On the other hand, there are more discussions in the literature about the rotational alignment of the tibial component.

Numerous anatomical landmarks have been described in the literature, including the medial third of the tibial tuberosity, the anterior tibial crest, the mid sulcus of tibia spine posterior tibial condylar line, the second ray, and the first web space of the foot. Aligning the tibial component to the tibial tubercle is one of the most popular landmark methods [7].

2. Tibia component landmarks in total knee arthroplasty

Many different landmarks have been studied to determine proper tibia component rotation, which can be divided into static and dynamic landmarks.

2.1 Static landmarks

Static landmarks can be divided into intraarticular references, which include anterior tibia crest, the posterior condylar line of the tibia, mid sulcus tibia spine, and the transcondylar line of the tibia, in some cases with extreme deformity, osteophytes formation, and tibia articular surface deficiency or unclear abnormal anatomy, which would make it difficult to visualize during surgery, and the conventional extraarticular landmarks references, such as transmalleolar axis and the axis of 2nd metatarsal bone, vary among patients and are not highly reliable as the various landmarks used. Therefore, various anatomic references have been proposed and used according to individual surgeons' preferences and experiences. These include Insall's reference, Akagi line, and posterolateral corner (curve on curve). Static landmarks may be affected by deformities like tibia torsion or foot pronation but are not affected by suboptimal femoral component rotation or poor soft tissue balancing.

2.1.1 Insall's reference

It is the most common landmark for tibia component rotation, first mentioned by Professor Insall in 1985 during his surgical technique of total knee replacement [8]. He aligned the tibia component to a fixation pin made centrally to the upper tibia at the medial third to the tibia tubercle toward the center of PCL tibia attachment (**Figure 1**).

2.1.2 Akagi line

The Akagi line is the line connecting the middle of PCL insertion at the tibia with the medial border of patellar tendon attachment (**Figure 2**) [9].

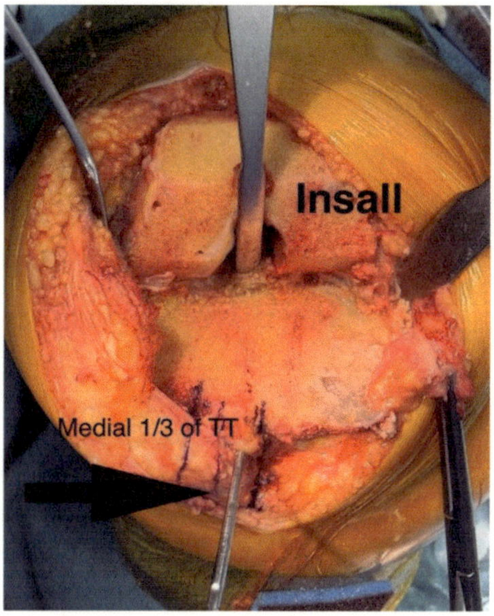

Figure 1.
Insall's Reference. Black arrow shows metal pin at the medial third of tibia tubercle projected toward the central point of the PCL insertion.

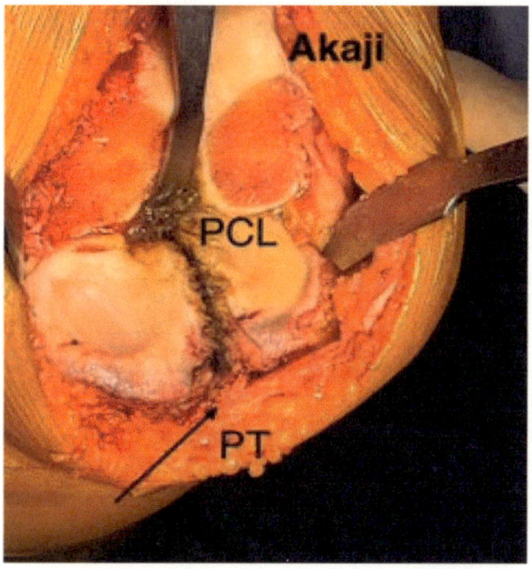

Figure 2.
Akagi Line. Medial border of patella ligament (arrow) to the center of tibia PCL insertion made just medial third of tibia tubercle).

2.1.3 The anterior Tibial cortex

MRI scan was done to align the anterior tibial cortex with the anterior tibia base plate [10]. The rotation was assessed in comparison to several landmarks. It was found that anterior tibial surface curvature is a more reliable and clearly recognizable landmark for tibial component alignment than other landmarks such as Akagi's line or medial third of tibial tubercle (**Figure 3**).

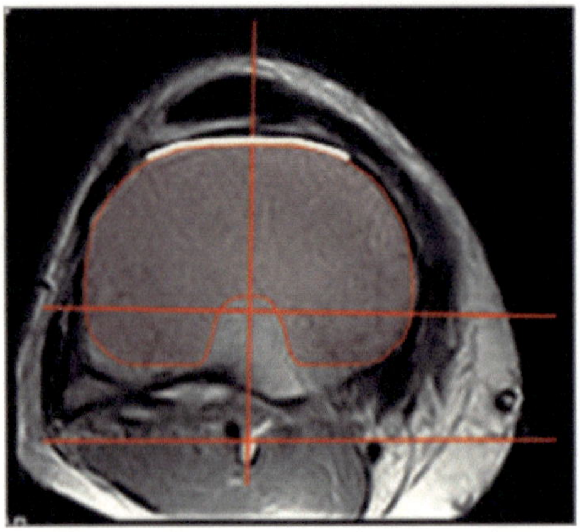

Figure 3.
Anterior medial cortex. MRI scan Tibial baseplate tracing superimposed on MRI matches anterior tibial cortex with anterior surface of baseplate; posteromedial corner not covered indicates sufficient external rotation of tibial component.

2.1.4 Mid sulcus tibia spine

Ozkan et al. described a technique in which the tibia component is aligned using the axis drawn from the center of the PCL to the sulcus between the tibial spines on the proximal tibia and to the tibialis anterior tendon at the ankle [11]. Postoperative CT scans done to assess coronal and axial alignment of the tibial component showed reliable alignment results.

2.1.5 Posterolateral corner (curve on curve)

The technique was introduced by Rossi et al. [12] in which the posterolateral corner of the proximal tibia is isolated and marked, then a trail tibia component tray with correct size should be aligned to match the posterolateral corner of the tibia without overhang and pinned, then the tibia base plate is externally rotated to match the anteromedial tibial cortex, and then fixed with a pin. The curve-on-curve method is easy but needs clear exposure of the lateral compartment of the knee to visualize the posterior-lateral corner of tibial plateau (**Figure 4**).

2.2 Kinematic techniques (self-seeking method/ROM/floating technique)

The self-seeking method aligns the tibial base plate according to the rotational alignment of the femoral component during trial reduction, after placing femoral and tibia trials and reducing patella multiple cycles of full extension, and flexion is performed [13].

Finally, the tibia component is marked with two pins.

The advantage of range of motion technique has been considered to represent the femorotibial kinematics. Additionally, many authors found that the ROM technique is not reliable to determine the tibia component rotation, as it carries the risk of transferring femoral malrotation to the tibia. Moreover, the position of the tibial tray is not solely determined by the femoral component. Instead, it's also influenced by several

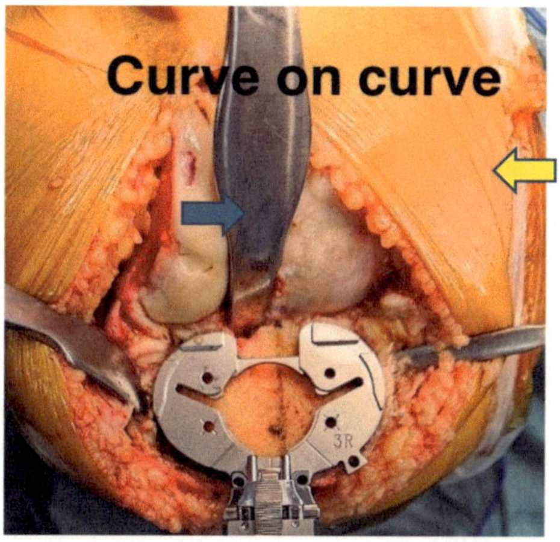

Figure 4.
Curve on curve technique. Posterolateral border is marked, and tibia component aligned (blue arrow) without overhang The tibia tray is then rotated externally until its anteromedial border to match the anteromedial border of the tibia (yellow arrow).

other factors, including the extensor mechanism, the patellar component, ligament balancing, and the tibial cut (**Figure 5**).

2.3 Maximizing tibial coverage to improve tibia rotation alignment

Anatomic designs provide better conformity, higher tibial coverage, more cortical support, lower incidence of downsizing, and less compromise of tibial coverage. Then proper rotational alignment is enforced, which improved tibial coverage and accuracy of rotational alignment. This design has significantly improved tibial component

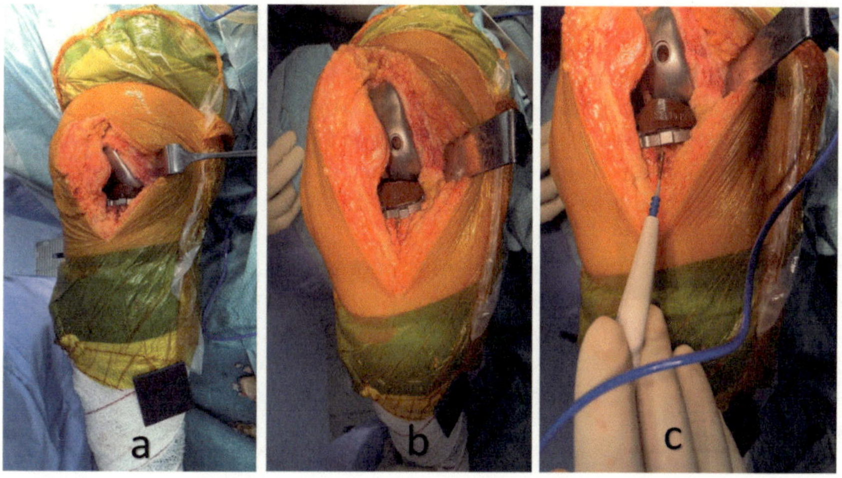

Figure 5.
ROM technique. (a) Trial components are fixed and knee in extension (b) multiple cycles of full extension and flexion performed. (c) Electrocautery used to mark anterior tibial component for rotational alignment.

internal malrotation, making it easier to balance rotation and coverage, thus leading to more effective and stable implant fixation [14, 15].

2.4 Computer-assisted navigation and robotic-assisted TKA

Advanced technology that has been used like computer-assisted navigation and robotic-assisted surgery has shown to improve accuracy of knee replacement surgery, but its future use is still under debate. Computer-assisted surgical navigation systems aims to improve implant alignment accuracy over traditional mechanical guides. However, this system relies on landmark digitization for rotational alignment that does not improve accuracy of rotational tibia alignment compared to traditional TKA instrumentation.

Robotic-assisted surgical technique used 3D-computed tomography (3DCT) measurements, superimposing preoperative plans onto postoperative images to directly compare prosthetic alignment. This technique significantly reduced outliers for rotational alignment of the tibial prosthesis compared to conventional TKA [16, 17].

3. Comparison between the most common landmarks currently used to determine the proper tibia rotation

Many authors have compared between the use of different static and kinematic tibia landmarks in order to investigate its effectiveness and reliability to determine a proper tibia rotation alignment.

In the study conducted by Chuan et al., they compared between the tibial-tubercle-landmark technique (TTL) and the range-of-motion technique (ROM). The TTL technique was found more prone to place the component in an externally rotated position compared with the ROM technique, but it still yielded good clinical outcomes. Due to variations in tibial tubercle anatomy and deformity, surgeons should master both methods and select the appropriate one based on specific conditions. Alternatively, both techniques could be used together to effectively reduce the incidence of rotational malalignment of the tibial component [18].

On the other hand, Ikeuchi et al. compared the ROM technique with the anatomical landmarks (Akaji references, tibia tubercle), and the result of their study showed significant difference of the tibial component rotation between the methods, since the ROM technique leads to more internally rotated tibial component than does the anatomical landmark one. Because of such wide variability and the several possibilities for error, they advised not to use the ROM technique as the sole method of determining alignment [19].

Elkabbani et al. compared the curve-on-curve technique with the ROM (free-floating technique) for tibial component, concluding that the curve-on-curve (anterior cortex referencing technique) places the tibial components in more external rotation compared to the free-floating technique. The anterior cortex referencing technique was found to be more reliable, and its use was recommended for early trained surgeons [20].

4. Measurements of tibial component rotation after TKA

Malrotation of the tibial component is linked with poor outcomes after TKA. The definition and evaluation of this problem remain debated due to inconsistent methods

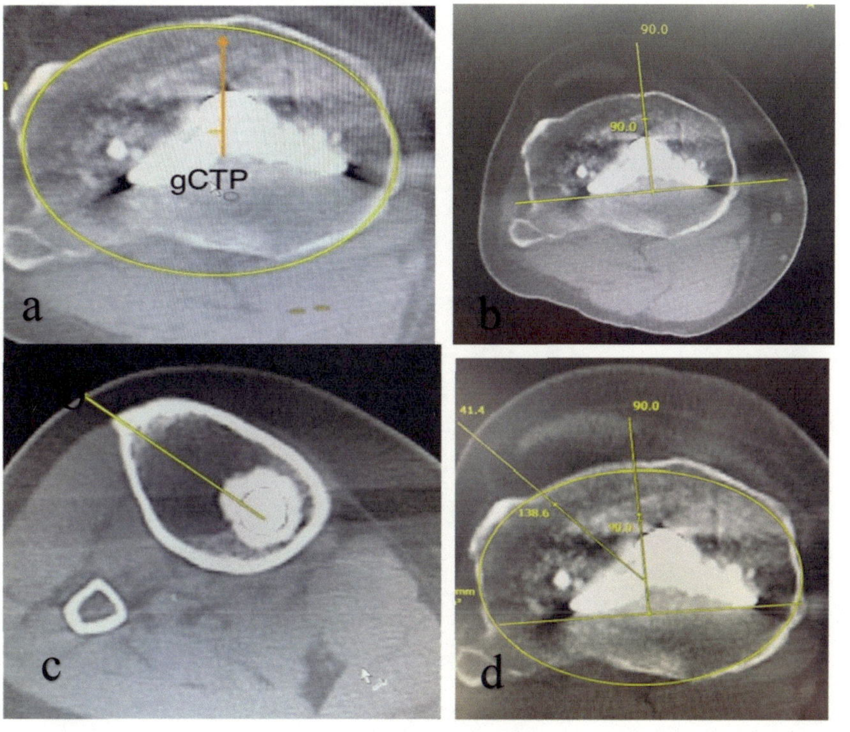

Figure 6.
The geometric center of the tibial plateau (gCTP) is the center of the best-fit circle of the proximal plateau. (b) The tibial component axis (TCA) is drawn as a perpendicular to a line connecting the posterior tibia component keel. (c) The tibial tubercle axis (TTA) is the line drawn from GCT to the most prominent part of the tubercle. (d) The tibia component rotation is the angle between TCA axis and TTA angle; in this case it shows 41.4, meaning the tibia component is internally rotated by more than 23 degrees relative to neutral tibia component rotation.

for measuring postoperative tibia component rotation. Several studies proposed measurement methods from which Berger et al. was the most commonly and most practically used one.

Berger measures tibia component rotation angle in the CT scan, which is the angle between the tibia component axis (TCA) and tibia tubercle axis (TAA). Normal rotation using this method is 18° (± 2.5°) internal rotation relative to the tip of tibia tubercle. Higher values indicate internal rotation of the tibial component relative to the tibial tubercle [21].

Berger et al. defined the tibia component axis as a line perpendicular to posterior condylar axis in symmetrical tibia designs. However, in modern asymmetrical tibia designs, we can use posterior tibia keel line (**Figure 6b**).

Elkabbani et al. have evaluated the tibial component rotation using MRI with metal artifact reduction for orthopedic implants (O-MAR). The technique has improved visualization of bone, implant-tissue interfaces, and periprosthetic soft tissue. Compared to CT scan, it adds more value to diagnose other findings and pain-causing complications of TKA that could be easily missed by CT scan, including polyethylene wear-induced synovitis and osteolysis metallosis, pseudo-tumors, fluid collections, periprosthetic joint infections, fracture, patellar clunk syndrome, recurrent hemarthrosis, arthrofibrosis, and ligamentous disruption. Similar technique as the Berger method is used to determine the tibial rotation (**Figure 7**) [22].

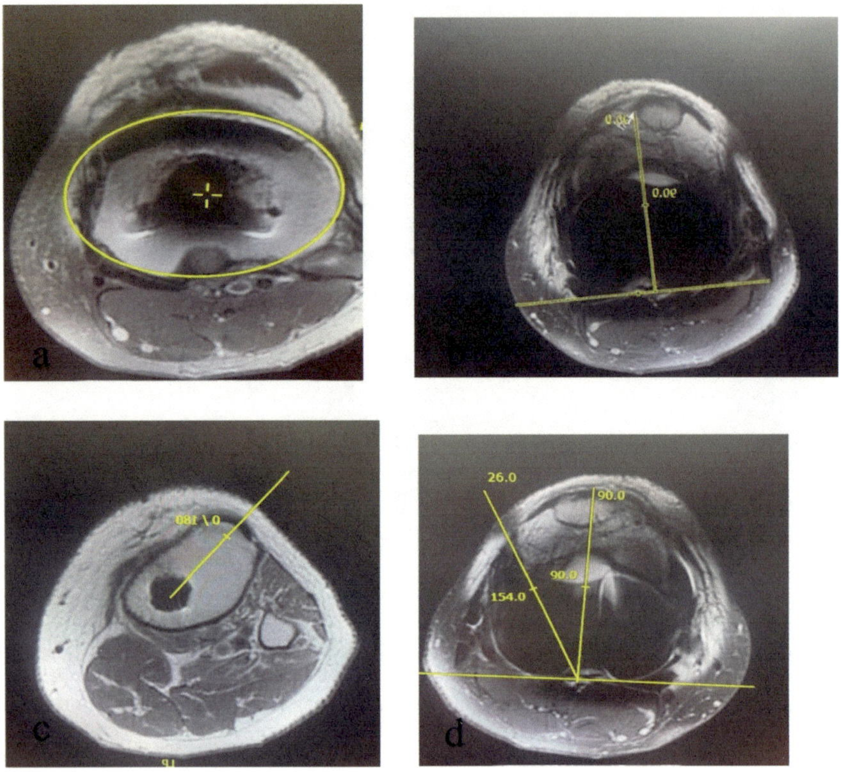

Figure 7.
(a,b,c) MRI images show similar technique to Berger methods used to determine the angle between the tibia component axis and tibia tubercle axis. (d) The angle is found to be 26 degrees, which indicates the internal tibia component rotation.

Picard et al. demonstrated a new landmark on the proximal tibia. He noticed that the lateral cortex of the tibia inferior to the tibia component was flat at a depth of approximately 10 mm from the joint line, the straightest line on a CT slice image (L) (**Figure 8**). A line can be drawn through the straightest part of the lateral tibial cortex, ignoring any osteophytes. A 2nd line perpendicular to this defined the reference axis (A). A line drawn through the posterior tibia component condyle represents the tibia component axis (B). The angle between A and B was measured to allow the rotation to be determined (**Figure 8**). Internal rotation was recorded as being negative and external rotation positive [23].

5. Clinical effects and potential complications associated of tibia component malrotation

Malalignment of the components has led to extension gap mismatch, also altering tibiofemoral kinematics and patellar maltracking. Because of these malalignments, they develop stiffness and chronic pain [24]. Ultimately, revision surgery will be needed to correct component malrotation [25].

The malrotation can disrupt the alignment between the tibial and femoral components, affecting patellar tracking. In addition, the severity of patellofemoral

DOI: http://dx.doi.org/10.5772/intechopen.1010394

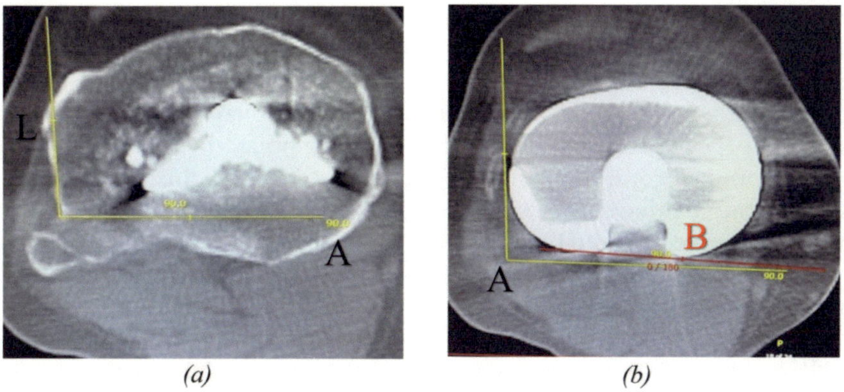

Figure 8.
(a) Measurement of tibial component rotation using the new landmark. The initial line (L) is aligned with the landmark of the straight lateral cortex of the tibia. A second line (A) drawn perpendicular to L defines the reference (anatomical) axis. (b) red line drawn through the posterior tibia component condyle represents the tibia component axis. The angle between A (yellow line) and B (red line) gives the tibial component rotation with internal rotation of the component (B with respect to A) being negative.

complications after TKA has been correlated with the amount of combined component internal rotation, as the internally rotated femoral component tightens the medial flexion gap, and the internally rotated tibial component has its posterolateral corner in a more anterior position. Given that posterior migration of the femoral condyle on the tibia with flexion occurs maximally in the lateral compartment, the internally rotated tibial component, especially of a conforming design, will limit rollback and flexion, leading to stiffness [24].

Many studies have linked the stiffness post knee replacement to the internal rotation of the tibia component. Abdelnasar et al. [24, 26] concluded that internal rotation of the tibial component in total knee arthroplasty (TKA) may contribute to postoperative extension deficits, resulting in pain and restricted motion. This issue arises because restricted external rotation of the tibial component can interfere with the "screw-home" mechanism, which is essential for achieving full knee extension. Combined with other previously discussed factors, this can ultimately lead to stiffness following TKA.

Tibia component malrotation can lead to increased wear and loosening as abnormal tibial rotation can cause uneven polyethylene wear, increasing the risk of early implant failure and osteolysis. Moreover, it can lead to progressive loosening of the tibial component, requiring revision surgery [26, 27].

The prosthetic component malrotation can accommodate only a limited range of rotational movement, typically between 2 and 8 degrees [26, 27].

6. Conclusion and recommendation

Total knee arthroplasty (TKA) is a largely successful procedure; however, malrotation of the prosthetic components has been linked to poor clinical outcomes. Therefore, ensuring proper rotation of the tibial component is a key surgical objective during TKA. Tibia component malrotation can lead to patellofemoral maltracking, increased wear, decreased range of motion, and an increased incidence of revision surgery. We recommend assessing the component rotation by CT scan using the

Berger method as a preoperative planning before revising total knee replacement especially in the case of patellofemoral malalignment, stiffness, or unexplained pain after primary knee replacement.

Too many intraarticular and extraarticular landmarks have been described in the literature. We believe that using the medial 1/3 of the tibial tubercle (Insall's reference), curve-on-curve and Akaji line is more accurate and reliable to determine tibia component rotation. Modern component designs have great effect on tibia rotation and coverage. We recommend the use of the asymmetrical (anatomical) tibia component designs, which can achieve the goals of tibial coverage, proper rotation, and minimal component overhang.

Up till now, the current literature has not identified a solid reliable anatomical landmark or a surgical technique that can ensure accurate rotational alignment of the tibial component in total knee arthroplasty. We anticipate that future advancements in technology, such as robotics, will enable precise determination of landmarks for tibial component rotation.

Author details

Muhammad Thahir[1,2], Ahmed Aly Naggar[1,2], Shaher Hasanain[1,2*], Mohamed Ragab[1,2], Alaa Aldeen Eydou[1,2], Abdul Sathar[1,2], Roshan Pais[1,2] and Khalid Al Hamadi[1,2]

1 Dubai Hospital, Dubai, United Arab Emirates

2 Mohammed Bin Rashid University of Medicine and Health Science, Dubai, United Arab Emirates

*Address all correspondence to: shaher1@hotmail.com

References

[1] Odum SM, Troyer JL, Kelly MP, Dedini RD, Bozic KJ. A cost-utility analysis comparing the cost-effectiveness of simultaneous and staged bilateral total knee arthroplasty. The Journal of Bone and Joint Surgery. American Volume. 2013;**95**:1441-1449

[2] Ranawat CS, Flynn WF, Saddler S, Hansraj KK, Maynard MJ. Long-term results of the total condylar knee arthroplasty. A 15-year survivorship study. Clinical Orthopaedics and Related Research. 2001;**388**:51-57

[3] Abdelnasser MK, Adi MM, Elnaggar AA, Tarabichi S. Internal rotation of the tibial component in total knee arthroplasty can lead to extension de cit. Knee Surgery, Sports Traumatology, Arthroscopy. 2020;**28**(9):2948-2952

[4] Eisenhuth SA, Saleh KJ, Cui Q, Clark CR, Brown TE. Patellofemoral instability after total knee arthroplasty. Clinical Orthopaedics and Related Research. 2006;**446**:149-160

[5] Luo CF. Reference axes for reconstruction of the knee. The Knee. 2004;**11**(4):251-257

[6] Benjamin J. Component alignment in total knee arthroplasty. Instructional Course Lectures. 2006;**55**:405-412

[7] Roper GE, Bloemke AD, Roberts CC, Spangehl MJ, Clarke HD. Analysis of tibial component rotation following total knee arthroplasty using 3D high definition computed tomography. The Journal of Arthroplasty. 2013;**28**(8 Suppl):106-111

[8] Insall JN, Binazzi R, Soudry M, Mestriner LA. Total knee arthroplasty. Clinical Orthopaedics and Related Research. 1985;**192**:13-22

[9] Akagi M, Oh M, Nonaka T, Tsujimoto H, Asano T, Hamanishi C. An anteroposterior axis of the tibia for total knee arthroplasty. Clinical Orthopaedics and Related Research. 2004;**420**:213-219. DOI: 10.1097/00003086-200403000-00030

[10] Dalury DF. Observations on proximal tibia in total knee arthroplasty. Clinical Orthopaedics and Related Research. 2001;**389**:150-155

[11] Sahin N, Atıcı T, Kurtoğlu Ü, Turgut A, Ozkaya G, Ozkan Y. Centre of posterior cruciate ligament & sulcus between tubercle spines are reliable landmarks for placement. Knee Surgery, Sports Traumatology, Arthroscopy. 2013;**21**(10):2384-2391

[12] Rossi R, Bruzzone M, Bonasia DE, et al. Evaluation of tibial rotational alignment in total knee arthroplasty: A cadaver study. Knee Surgery, Sports Traumatology, Arthroscopy. 2010;**18**:889-893. DOI: 10.1007/s00167-009-1023-6

[13] Ikeuchi M, Yamanaka N, Okanoue Y, Ueta E, Tani T. Determining the rotational alignment of the tibial component at total knee replacement: A comparison of two techniques. Journal of Bone and Joint Surgery. British Volume (London). 2007;**89**(1):45-49. DOI: 10.1302/0301-620X.89B1.17728

[14] Dai Y, Scuderi GR, Bischoff JE, Bertin K, Tarabichi S, Rajgopal A. Anatomic tibial component design can increase tibial coverage and rotational alignment accuracy: A comparison of six contemporary designs. Knee Surgery,

Sports Traumatology, Arthroscopy. 2014;**22**(12):2911-2923. DOI: 10.1007/s00167-014-3282-0. Epub 2014 Sep 13

[15] Martin S, Saurez A, Ismaily S, Ashfaq K, Noble P, Incavo SJ. Maximizing tibial coverage is detrimental to proper rotational alignment. Clinical Orthopaedics and Related Research. 2014;**472**(1):121-125. DOI: 10.1007/s11999-013-3047-y

[16] Siston RA, Goodman SB, Patel JJ, Delp SL, Giori NJ. The high variability of tibial rotational alignment in total knee arthroplasty. Clinical Orthopaedics and Related Research. 2006;**452**:65-69. DOI: 10.1097/01.blo.0000229335.36900.a0

[17] Kuriyama S, Hyakuna K, Inoue S, Tamaki Y, Ito H, Matsuda S. Tibial rotational alignment was significantly improved by use of a CT-navigated control device in total knee arthroplasty. The Journal of Arthroplasty. 2014;**29**(12):2352-2356. DOI: 10.1016/j.arth.2014.06.016. Epub 2014 Jun 28

[18] Liu Xin MS, Mao Xingjia MD, Guo Shengjie MS, Cao Yanwei MD, Li Shuaijie MD, Xiang Chuan MD. Comparison of tibial tubercle landmark technique and range of motion technique in primary Total knee arthroplasty: A retrospective cohort study. Orthopaedic Surgery. 2022;**14**:3159-3170. DOI: 10.1111/os.13486

[19] Ikeuchi M, Yamanaka N, Okanoue Y, Ueta E, Tani T. Determining the rotational alignment of the tibial component at total knee replacement. Journal of Bone and Joint Surgery (British). 2007;**89-B**:45-49. DOI: 10.1302/0301-620X.89B1

[20] Elkabbani M, Saied AM, Abouelnas BA, Dragos A, Osman A, Tarabichi S. Curve-on-curve technique is more reliable than free-floating technique for tibial components positioning in posterior stabilized total knee arthroplasty using symmetrical tibial components in varus osteoarthritis. BMC Musculoskeletal Disorders. 2024;**25**:1009. DOI: 10.1186/s12891-024-07975-0

[21] Berger RA, Crossett LS, Jacobs JJ, Rubash HE. Malrotation causing patellofemoral complications after total knee arthroplasty. Clinical Orthopaedics and Related Research. 1998;**356**:144-153. DOI: 10.1097/00003086-199811000-00021

[22] Elkabbani M, Osman AA, Helaly M, Tarabichi S. Evaluation of tibial component rotation in painful total knee arthroplasties by MRI enhanced with metal artifact reduction technique. Journal of Musculoskeletal Research (BMC Musculoskeletal Disorders). 2024;**25**:1009. DOI: 10.1142/s0218957721500123

[23] Mahmood FF, Holloway NJ, Deakin AH, Clarke JV, Picard F. A new landmark for measuring tibial component rotation after total knee arthroplasty. The Knee. 2019;**26**(3):779-786

[24] Abdelnasser MK, Adi MM, Elnaggar AA, Tarabichi S. Internal rotation of the tibial component in total knee arthroplasty can lead to extension deficit. Knee Surgery, Sports Traumatology, Arthroscopy. 2020;**28**(9):2948-2952

[25] Baker PN, Van der Meulen JH, Lewsey J, Gregg PJ. The role of pain and function in determining patient satisfaction after total knee replacement: Data from the National Joint Registry for England and Wales. Journal of Bone and Joint Surgery. British Volume

(London). 2007;**89-B**:893-900. DOI: 10.1302/0301-620X.89B7.19091

[26] Kim HY, Kim KJ, Yang DS, Jeung SW, Choi HG, Choy WS. Screw-home movement of the tibiofemoral joint during normal gait: Three-dimensional analysis. Clinics in Orthopedic Surgery. 2015;7:303-309

[27] Nicoll D, Rowley DI. Internal rotational error of the tibial components is a major cause of pain after total knee replacement. Journal of Bone and Joint Surgery. British Volume (London). 2010;**92-B**:1238-1244. DOI: 10.1302/0301-620X.92B9.23516

Chapter 3

Infection in Total Joint Arthroplasty: Has the Technology Improved Diagnosis and Management?

Varun Narula, Sumit Anand, Ravindra Mohan and Devang Bharti

Abstract

Total joint arthroplasty enhances patients' well-being by reconstructing joints to thereby restoring mobility and alleviating pain. However, the problem of infections cuts down recovery time while burdening medical facilities. This chapter showcases the transformative impact of modern technological advancements on infection diagnosis and treatment methods. The current standards for diagnosis utilize clinical evaluations, serum marker detection, synovial fluid exams, and imaging tests to establish infections. These are complemented by treatments of debridement with prosthesis retention, one-stage or two-stage revisions, and systemic antibiotic therapy. Modern technology extends detection methods by implementing rapid biomarkers of synovial fluid, molecular diagnostics, and next-generation sequencing techniques. They bring high-resolution imaging technology and artificial intelligence support for enhanced and faster infection discovery. Orthopedic infection management is enhanced through combined revision surgery procedures and enhanced irrigation procedures and localized antibiotic administration systems, as well as resistant bacteriophage treatment and antimicrobial-infused implants. Faster analysis is enabled through the advanced technology as it speeds up infection removal as well as minimizing the patients' recovery duration, thereby ending prior health setbacks owing to treatment. Their efficiency is compromised through elevated costs as well as inadequate proof of advancements, meeting with varied regional patient access obstacles. This chapter reviews changing infection-control methods in total joint arthroplasty through comparisons of innovative technological care products.

Keywords: total joint arthroplasty, diagnostic technology, infection management, synovial biomarkers, molecular diagnostics, revision surgery, antimicrobial implants

1. Introduction

Total joint arthroplasty (TJA) is an important orthopedic surgery where surgeons provide functional rehabilitation benefits along with relief of pain for patients suffering from severe joint ailments. It is mostly undertaken as hip and knee replacement surgery in patients suffering from arthritis and severe degenerative joint disease. It has become an integral practice in the medical field due to the emphasis being placed on active lifestyle in the elderly population, leading to higher yearly procedure volume. Infection is, however, still an inherent problem in total joint arthroplasty, manifesting mostly as joint infection complications. These infections become challenges toward successful outcomes within constraints, having a significant impact on the patient outcome and on the healthcare system.

The strength of TJA is that it can replace a damaged joint with a prosthetic, allowing patients to regain lost function. Hip and knee replacements account for most of these procedures, and hundreds of thousands of people in the United States alone [1]. Its scale indicates both the acceptance of the procedure and the size of the quality-of-life boost it provides. If infection takes a grip, patients face significant setbacks. Many suffer severe pain, frequently joined by swelling and stiffness that erases gains in mobility that TJA attempts to restore. The economic cost is also astronomical, reaching tens of thousands of dollars per case, a burden that increases as TJA becomes increasingly common.

Infections in joint arthroplasty occur when bacteria infest the prosthetic joint, often forming a protective biofilm that shields them from immune defense and therapeutic strategies. This characteristic makes identification and eradication incredibly challenging. Surgeons have had a problem in reliably identifying these infections over decades without any single definitive test. Diagnosis rests on a combination of clinical presentation, laboratory results, and imaging. Open sinus tracts or recurring positive cultures provide firm evidence, but many cases lack this clear-cut indicator. Some infections resist detection using routine cultures, obscuring the diagnostic process [2]. Treatment may involve surgical interventions, ranging from joint washing to complete prosthesis removal, in combination with protracted antibiotic therapy. Results are variable, often requiring repeated procedures and resulting in lengthy recovery or permanent disability.

In total joint arthroplasty, infection has the greatest effect on a per-procedure basis. Orthopedic surgeons regard TJA as central to their practice, but infection undermines their capacity for achieving permanent outcomes. Accurate diagnosis can contain infection, but delays can compound the problem. Treatment options weigh eradication of infection against preservation of joint function, directly dictating outcomes for the patient [3]. Patients bear the burden of these complications, as infection disrupts the relief of pain and mobility that TJA has the potential to deliver, extending their discomfort for months. Greater frequency of TJA, with changing demographics and increasing indications for surgery, heightens the urgency to address this issue.

Technological advancements are on the verge of streamlining the diagnosis and management of infection in total joint arthroplasty. New technology and tools emerge periodically to enable enhanced detection at onset, better detection of pathogens, and enhanced eradication of infection. These advancements hold the key to improving outcomes for orthopedic surgeons who want to optimize the outcomes of TJA, as well as for patients who want proper recuperation [3]. Increased TJA use increases the need for establishing whether such advancements indeed impact joint replacement care, an area of concern for both clinical practice and the patient experience.

DOI: http://dx.doi.org/10.5772/intechopen.1010881

2. Current standard for management

2.1 Diagnosis

Total joint arthroplasty relies on meticulous diagnosis to retain its position as a cutting-edge procedure in orthopedics, especially in joint replacements in which infection can nullify clinical success. It is preceded by thorough clinical evaluation, the key first step toward identifying impending infection in TJA. The joint is examined by surgeons for pain that does not resolve within normal postoperative periods, as reported by the patient. Fever may be present with these results, but its absence does not exclude infection, particularly in chronic infection with muted sequelae. These results may be confused with aseptic complications (e.g., implant wear, periprosthetic fracture) and, as such, have dictated a step-wise approach for diagnosis [4]. Laboratory evaluations and imaging studies are adjuncts that create a body of evidence that has bio-objective findings on which to distinguish infection from other complications in TJA. This approach is sequential and mechanistic and forms a framework for surgeons to reliably diagnose problems in total joint arthroplasty, ensuring timely treatment or a safeguard for patient outcomes.

Serum biomarkers are a useful screening tool in total joint arthroplasty. Biomarkers provide color regarding the amount of systemic inflammation present in the TJA, for example, in difficult joint replacement patients. The erythrocyte sedimentation rate and C-reactive protein levels are requested routinely and are general indicators of the body's reaction to potential infection. Postsurgical normal elevation makes early assessment tricky, with erythrocyte sedimentation rate (ESR) frequently over 30 millimeters per hour and C-reactive protein (CRP) over 10 milligrams per liter in the initial month following TJA, even in the absence of infection [5]. Specificity fails in autoimmune conditions, recent trauma, or infection in some other location, and surgeons need to interpret results in this regard. White cell count is used in addition in some cases, though in TJA, leukocytosis is less sensitive and often remains normal until the infection is severe. These markers serve as a gateway, flagging cases for further examination in the management of total joint arthroplasty.

Synovial analysis provides a window closer to the condition of the prosthetic joint in total joint arthroplasty and is hence a staple of infection diagnosis in joint replacements. Fluid is aspirated by surgeons under sterile conditions, usually under the guidance of ultrasound or fluoroscopy, where anatomy makes it tricky in the hip [6]. Leukocyte levels greater than 3000 cells per microliter with many polymorphonuclear neutrophils indicate acute infection. In comparison, chronic infections fall to 1500 cells per microliter and more than half of neutrophils, indicative of a less acute inflamed process. Immediate bacteria can be glimpsed with Gram stain, albeit its low sensitivity teeters, which restricts its usefulness. Cultures are grown for at least 5 days—up to 14 days for slow growers like *Cutibacterium acnes*—in an attempt to find the causative pathogen. Pre-inciting antibiotic ingestion, even a single dose, can impede growth and result in some cases of false negatives [7]. Re-aspiration after a drug holiday enhances yield, a strategy catching acceptance in TJA. Its direct analysis is still invaluable, linking the suspects to actionable microbial data.

Imaging modalities fill in the diagnostic picture of total joint arthroplasty infection, providing functional and structural information concerning joint prostheses. Plain radiographs, taken in both anteroposterior and lateral projections, are the entry point, showing periosteal elevation, focal osteolysis, or loosening of the implant indicative of infection. They are too insensitive in early infection to allow them to be used in any capacity other than ruling out gross abnormalities, and evidence of bone loss occurring rapidly over weeks rather than months poses red flags [7]. Computed tomography scans define soft tissue extension, locating abscesses, sinus tracts, or peri-implant collections of fluid, although metal artifacts of the prosthesis degrade images and require sophisticated reconstruction algorithms [8]. Magnetic resonance imaging is superior in depicting marrow edema or osteomyelitis, optimized by metal suppression sequences to overcome implant interference. Nuclear scanning, for example, technetium-99m bone scans and indium-111 leukocyte scans, detects infection by locating sites of increased metabolism with a high sensitivity but is compromised by low specificity due to aseptic inflammation or prior surgery. Positron emission tomography using fluorodeoxyglucose provides a higher definition in selected centers, although cost and availability restrict it to routine application. Together, these modalities sharpen the picture of infection in TJA, filling gaps in clinical and laboratory examination.

2.2 Treatment

Total joint infection requires an aggressive, tailored approach that optimizes joint replacement with the combination of antimicrobial treatment and meticulous surgery. Timing is the determinant of the approach. For instance, acute infection within few weeks post-surgery favors conservative management, while chronic infection elicited over months requires major reconstruction. Patient-specific factors of age, comorbidities, and bone stock impact decision-making, as do implant stability, intraoperatively or with imaging. Overall objectives balance infection cure with preservation of joint function, a delicate equation constituting today's TJA standards. Surgeons move across a continuum of options, each defined by separate protocols, results, and difficulties, optimizing individualized care for the patient in whom this complication arises in total joint arthroplasty.

Debridement, antibiotics, and implant retention (DAIR) is a joint-preserving approach to acute infection in total joint arthroplasty. It addresses infections that occur in the first 6 weeks after index joint replacement or by hematogenous seeding, frequently of oral or urinary origin. Surgeons approach the joint by the original incision and remove infected synovium, necrotic tissue, and hematoma and then irrigate three to nine liters of normal saline, occasionally added to by povidone-iodine or chlorhexidine for additional antimicrobial kick [9]. Modular components of polyethylene liners are removed to break up biofilm, and the fixed prosthesis is retained if well anchored. Intravenous vancomycin or ceftriaxone for broad antimicrobial protection starts intraoperatively and lasts 6 to 8 weeks, based on cultures or empiric therapy if cultures are negative. Single-stage simplicity is the strength of DAIR, although failure necessitates revision surgery, a standard step in infection management of TJA.

Two-step revision prevails as the gold standard for chronic infection in total joint arthroplasty, where its painstakingness commands confidence. Stage one mobilizes the infected joint prosthesis, a meticulous process that includes cement extraction, complete debridement of all cement-coated bone and soft tissue, and copious irrigation to remove lingering bacteria. An antibiotic-loaded spacer, frequently static in knees or articulating in hips, is modeled in polymethylmethacrylate cement polymerized with antibiotics such as vancomycin and tobramycin, providing local concentrations of drug 1000-fold higher than systemic levels. Patients immobilize the joint for weeks using crutches or immobilization, while intravenous antibiotics—specific to microorganisms on occasion, such as *Staphylococcus epidermidis* or gram-negatives—cycle for 6 to 12 weeks, tracked by ESR, CRP, and wound healing [10]. Stage 2, 3 to 6 months later, when infection markers normalize and aspirate, yields sterility, substitutes a new prosthesis, and frequently uses antibiotic-loaded cement for adjunct prophylaxis. Cure rates reach high levels, although spacer complications (dislocation, fracture) or recurrence in some patients prolong the ordeal [10]. While intensity makes the modality laborious, reliability establishes it as a pillar of TJA infection management.

One-stage revision is an efficient alternative for infection in total joint arthroplasty and is popular in Europe for appropriate joint cases. Surgeons perform the procedure in one sitting—removing the offending prosthesis, thoroughly debriding to healthy bleeding tissue, lavaging by pulsed irrigation, and replacing the prosthesis with antibiotic-burdened cement, frequently gentamicin or dual-drug loading. Candidates are those with known flora by preoperative aspirate, soft tissue quality, and adequate bone stock to accept immediate fixation. Six to twelve weeks of intravenous antibiotics follow, shorter in a few programs, taking advantage of high local drug concentrations to sweep up lingering bacteria. Cure rates are comparable to two-stage procedures with the advantages of fewer complications, one anesthetic experience, and quicker recovery to function possibly in 3 months [11]. Reinfection risks remain if debridement fails to encompass clinically concealed bacteria in resistance-inducing crevices, requiring surgical skill and strict patient selection. This strategy makes headway in TJA, securing efficacy without compromising the economy.

Antibiotic therapy secures infection treatment in TJA, magnifying the impact of surgery in joint replacement. Prophylactic antibiotics, usually cefazolin (1–2 grams) or vancomycin (15 milligrams per kilogram) in the case of penicillin allergy, are infused precisely 60 minutes and dosed every 4 hours in the case of lengthy TJA procedures to ensure tissue levels remain above the minimum inhibitory concentration [7]. Intravenous administration is the rule for 2 to 6 weeks, followed by oral agents such as levofloxacin or linezolid for outpatient, finishing for 8 to 12 weeks. Local antibiotics placed in cement or beads, charged with 2 to 4 grams of drug per 40-gram load, reach synovial concentrations far over systemic dosing, maximizing outcomes without incurring much toxicity in the form of renal impairment or ototoxicity monitored by lab testing. This dual-track approach maximizes infection protection in TJA, balancing specificity with pragmatism.

2.3 Prevention

Infection prevention in total joint arthroplasty remains a linchpin of success, particularly in joint replacement, where complications cascade through life and healthcare systems. Current practices spin a close web of preoperative, intraoperative, and postoperative steps, each aimed against specific infection routes. Patient optimization addresses individual risk, operating room technique stops contamination, and follow-up watchfulness protects the recovering joint. An all-around effort mirrors the high stakes of TJA in preemption of the intensive therapy described previously by keeping infection away in the first place.

Preoperative optimization focuses on individualized vulnerabilities before initiating total joint arthroplasty. Surgeons examine body mass index, prompting patients over 40 kilograms per square meter to lose weight to reduce infection risk. Fat tissue impedes wound closure and immune function in joint arthroplasty [12, 13]. Diabetes management focuses on insulin titration or dietary instruction over a few months, normalizing blood glucose to support healing. Smoking cessation, instituted 4 to 8 weeks prior to operation by nicotine patches or counseling, turns off vasoconstriction and enhances tissue oxygen supply. Nasal swab testing for *Staphylococcus aureus* prompts carriers to be treated using the application of mupirocin ointment for 5 days and daily bathing in chlorhexidine, which halves infection risk in some groups. Immunosuppressive medications, such as methotrexate in rheumatoid arthritis or chronic steroids, are halted or weaned under specialist direction [12]. Malnutrition screening by albumin levels less than 3.5 grams per deciliter should trigger protein supplementation, thus increasing success rates of TJA.

Intraoperative prevention constructs a sterile barrier during total joint arthroplasty, keeping bacteria away from joint prostheses. Operating rooms use laminar airflow or ultraclean ventilation, reducing most airborne microbes in conjunction with positive pressure to keep contaminants away. Surgeons then wear sterile gowns, hoods, and two pairs of gloves (replaced if penetrated); skin preparation using chlorhexidine-alcohol surpasses that of iodine in efficacy, drying completely before draping, and flushing the joint with 3 to 6 liters of saline. Antibiotic cement, releasing 1 to 2 grams of gentamicin per batch, encapsulates primary implants in high-risk cases or all revisions, releasing the drug for weeks [14]. Abbreviated operating times and limited door openings finish this fortress, keeping TJA from infection's reign.

Postoperative prevention extends these efforts beyond the operating room in total joint arthroplasty, bolstering joint recoveries. Wounds are given occlusive dressings for 48 to 72 hours, replaced only if soaked, with silver-impregnated dressings in some protocols to inhibit bacterial growth. Surgeons examine incisions for 48 hours, then palpate for heat, induration, or purulent discharge weekly, escalating to aspiration if suspected. Patients are taught to dry sites, avoiding baths or pools for 3 weeks until the wound is sealed by epithelialization and fortified by suture or staple removal at 14 to 21 days. Antibiotic prophylaxis for dental procedures or colonoscopies, usually 2 grams of amoxicillin 1 hour in advance, blocks hematogenous seeding 2 years post-TJA or lifelong in high-risk populations such as diabetics [14]. Follow-ups in 2, 6 weeks, 3 months, and annually monitor joint health by exam and X-rays, with lab orders of the type of CRP for persistent pain. Extended vigilance in this way detects infections in the TJA surface early, saving the gains of the procedure.

3. Recent advancements and technological improvements

3.1 Diagnostic innovations

Recent advancements in diagnosing infections in total joint arthroplasty have introduced cutting-edge tools that elevate the care of joint replacements beyond what was possible a decade ago. These advances are important because early detection and identification of infections can change the course of treatment in TJA entirely. Surgeons today depend on technologies that surpass previous methods in speed and accuracy, lessening the guesswork associated with infection management. Patients undergoing joint replacement benefit from expedited answers that equate to expedited treatments and less danger of joint damage. The impetus of these technologies is to keep infections from silently eroding the success of total joint arthroplasty [15]. Diagnostic tools that address the specific challenge of prosthetic joints, where biofilms and subtle symptoms conceal the issue, are emerging. This results from a more significant movement in orthopedics to optimize the detection and identification of infections in TJA.

Synovial fluid biomarkers are taking center stage as a game-changer in total joint arthroplasty diagnostics, providing surgeons with a fast and dependable method of infection detection in joint replacements. Alpha-defensin testing is in the lead, using a protein that neutrophils release in response to the presence of bacteria. In stark contrast to days or weeks, it yields results in a few hours for the cultures to mature. It excels in that antibiotics do not skew its results, a usual pitfall for conventional methods. Data indicate high sensitivity, providing surgeons with confidence in the outcome. Calprotectin becomes a strong biomarker in support, measuring inflammation directly in the synovial fluid extracted from the joint [15]. It often keeps pace with alpha-defensin but is less expensive, providing a cost-efficient alternative to deploy in more significant numbers. Leukocyte esterase, borrowed from humble dipstick assays, offers a reliable bedside alternative. These biomarkers equip clinicians with means of nailing infections quickly, informing treatment plans for TJA with greater clarity than ever.

Pathogen identification in total joint arthroplasty has come of age thanks to molecular diagnostics, which bring a level of specificity that changes the game for surgeons managing joint infection. Next-generation sequencing is unique in looking for bacteria in extracted DNA, synovial fluid, or tissue specimens removed during the operation. It detects bacteria that get by standard cultures, particularly low-virulence bugs such as *Cutibacterium acnes* or unusual gram-negatives. It is particularly strong in culture-negative infections, which account for a quarter of cases of TJA, successfully identifying pathogens in many challenging cases [16]. It takes 1 or 2 days for results, saving critical days of diagnostic lag versus the 5 to 14 days that cultures may require. Matrix-assisted laser desorption/ionization time-of-flight mass spectrometry gains speed on another front. It reads bacterial protein in positive cultures, identifying species minutes after growth is seen. Polymerase chain reaction assays amplify joint samples' bacterial DNA, providing same-day detection of typical TJA pathogens such as *Staphylococcus aureus*. These molecular technologies allow surgeons to see infection in tight focus faster, improving the chances of successful management in total joint arthroplasty.

Imaging technologies have made giant leaps forward to support infection diagnosis in total joint arthroplasty, giving better images of what is happening in and around joint prostheses. Metal artifact reduction sequence magnetic resonance imaging addresses the distortion introduced by implants, a longtime imaging TJA challenge. It discloses soft tissue changes such as synovial hyperplasia, fluid collections, or sinus tracts that show infection, approaching very high sensitivity levels. When combined with bone marrow scanning, white blood cell scintigraphy refines specificity compared to dated nuclear technologies like technetium bone scans. It screens out aseptic inflammation versus infection in joints, reducing the false positives [16]. Positron emission tomography using fluorodeoxyglucose raises the bar again with high-definition images of the hotspots of metabolism. It marks infection sites correctly, often identifying bone involvement that X-rays miss. Single-photon emission computed tomography combines nuclear and CT data for a 3D perspective, assisting surgeons in gauging infection depth in TJA [13]. These imaging advances inform surgical planning, ensuring treatments find their mark in total joint arthroplasty.

Artificial intelligence is prominent in total joint arthroplasty diagnosis, improving how infections are detected in joint replacements. Machine learning programs comb through sinuous amounts of data like lab reports, imaging, and patient history to predict the likelihood of infection. These models learn to identify subtle markers, such as faint periosteal reactions or biomarker patterns that might escape human eyes on their own [17]. Artificial intelligence interoperates with electronic health records, identifying high-risk joint patients in real time with alerts for the surgeon. Some configurations complement synovial fluid analysis, correlating levels of alpha-defensin with imaging to increase confidence. Others compare serial X-rays after TJA, following changes over weeks to identify creeping infections. Artificial intelligence is serving as a second set of eyes, improving diagnosis and accelerating total joint arthroplasty care.

Point-of-care testing has taken diagnostics to the bedside in total joint arthroplasty, a quantum leap in controlling joint infection. Point-of-care devices now quantify synovial biomarkers such as alpha-defensin or leukocyte esterase in a few milliliters of joint aspirate. Results appear in less than 20 minutes, a far cry from laboratory turnaround times of several hours or days. They are as accurate as lab assays, with a very high sensitivity [17]. Surgeons can perform them in a clinic during a follow-up visit or even in the OR amid the procedure, confirming infection in real time. Some devices complement smartphone apps, storing data for instant assessment. Immediacy reduces the waiting time between suspicion and intervention, a critical advantage in TJA, where each hour is important in joint salvage.

3.2 Management innovations

Management of infections in total joint arthroplasty has leaped forward with technological improvements, giving surgeons fresh ways to tackle joint infections head-on. These advances seek to eradicate bacteria better while preserving the joint functional in patients. Surgical tricks, drug delivery systems, and implant designs that have come out in the last decade reduce the painstaking repeat procedures that previously characterized infection care in TJA. Patients experience shorter in-hospital stays and improved opportunities for return to everyday life. These steps strongly reflect wiser, more judicious infection management in total joint arthroplasty.

Surgical methods in total joint arthroplasty have improved with the advent of the 1.5-stage revision, a hybrid alternative to joint infection. Surgeons begin by removing the infected prosthesis, scraping away all the infected tissue, and cleaning the joint in one sitting. They then implant an articulating spacer full of antibiotics such as vancomycin or gentamicin, allowing the patient to mobilize the hip or knee as the antibiotics get to work in 6 to 12 weeks. The design of the spacer approximates a natural joint, and it protects muscle tone and range—often, patients can bear weight using the walker in a few days [18]. Later, a follow-up operation replaces the space with a lifelong prosthesis when no infection is in sight, according to laboratory tests and aspirations. Such a configuration eradicates most infections, comparable to two-stage revision, without putting patients through the extensive immobilization of static spacers. It combines efficiency and function, a significant victory in TJA recovery.

Irrigation solutions significantly upgraded total joint arthroplasty, enhancing how surgeons clean out joint infections. Acetic acid solutions, diluted to clinically safe concentrations, attack biofilms during debridement, breaking down the adhesive layers that protect bacteria from antibiotics. Polymeric irrigants infused with antimicrobial peptides escalate it further [19]. These liquids adhere to joint surfaces, releasing bactericides for many postoperative hours, reaching regions where standard washing fails. Some preparations introduce surfactants to disintegrate debris, clearing the arena for healing. Pulsed lavage systems are now used by surgeons to blast these solutions in, pushing them deep into bone and tissue. These developments make infection clearance in TJA harder for bacteria to avoid.

Antibiotic delivery systems have leveled up in total joint arthroplasty, delivering drugs directly where they are needed in joint infections. The VT-X7 delivers vancomycin or ceftriaxone directly into the joint via a small catheter driven by a wearable device [18]. It sustains drug levels stratospheric—up to 10,000 micrograms per milliliter—for days, far surpassing what IV drips can achieve without putting a strain on the kidneys. Calcium sulfate beads provide another twist, sculpted with antibiotics like tobramycin intraoperatively. They break down in 4 to 6 weeks, releasing drugs into the joint, then disappear without a follow-up operation. Some surgeons combine them with cement spacers for a 1–2 punch. These systems attack infections aggressively in TJA, closing the gap that antibiotics cannot.

Bacteriophage therapy emerged as a biological remedy for total joint arthroplasty infection, attacking joint cases in precision strikes. Phages are viruses that chase specific bacteria, administered in the joint during the procedure or through catheters afterward. They disintegrate biofilms and hard-to-treat bugs like methicillin-resistant *Staphylococcus aureus*, where antibiotics lose their way. Preliminary application in TJA demonstrates high clearance rates, frequently in combination with standard medications, without harming human cells [20]. Phage cocktails are customized in the laboratory to match individualized patient cultures, a perfect pairing where some centers maintain ready-to-administer phage collections for everyday pathogens. It is well-tolerated by the patient population, and there are no significant side effects to report yet. It introduces a living tool to the TJA toolbox, attacking infections that baffle conventional treatments.

Implant technologies have introduced new infection defenses in total joint arthroplasty, bolstering joint replacements from day 1. Prosthetics coated in silver discharge ions that kill bacteria upon contact were tested in infection-prone patients such as diabetics or revision cases. Antibiotic-bonded implants form chemical bonds to attach drugs such as gentamicin to the top, seeping away over weeks to prevent adhesion. Tests in the lab show that bacterial levels fall by 99% near these devices. Photocatalytic coatings, activated by UV light in the OR, spit out oxygen radicals that sterilize the implant for several hours after placement [20]. Some prototypes combine silver with ceramics, doubling the protection. These technologies bring a built-in defense to TJA, reducing infection odds on the front end.

Risk assessment systems have tapped technology to identify danger in advance in total joint arthroplasty. Predictive models crunch data—age, BMI, diabetes, and history of smoking, and previous TJA—before surgery, spitting out infection risk scores for joint patients. Machine learning refines these systems, folding in real-time statistics such as OR time or post-op wound drainage patterns [18]. Some systems follow patients after discharge through apps, flagging fevers or redness for early clinic appointments. These models translate guesswork to strategy, shaving infection rates in TJA by identifying threats ahead of the curve.

Intraoperative diagnostics have introduced real-time information to total joint arthroplasty, revolutionizing how joint infections are managed in the operating room. Implants of portable polymerase chain reaction units check tissue or fluid samples for bacterial DNA during a procedure, often identifying pathogens in less than 1 hour. This allows surgeons to adjust antibiotics such as substituting cefazolin for vancomycin or lengthen debridement on the fly. Digitized frozen section histology scans tissue slices for neutrophils, which pathologists interpret remotely in minutes. It is susceptible to excluding active infection and determining whether to reimplant that day. Some centers supplement it with rapid biomarker testing, measuring alpha-defensin levels intra-op. These technologies make the operating room a diagnostic center, increasing the success of TJA.

3.3 Evidence of improvement

Emerging technologies bring clear victories in treating infection in total joint arthroplasty, remediating overall outcomes in joint replacement. Diagnosis zeroes in on infections today, whereas treatments strike harder and quicker. Patients experience it with fewer setbacks and briefer recoveries. Surgeons encounter fewer challenging cases. Data mounts that these tools are effective, though challenges remain. These advances are directly related to actual changes in TJA care.

Diagnostic enhancements in total joint arthroplasty reduce delays and increase confidence for joint infections. Synovial biomarkers such as alpha-defensin reduces wait days to hours, and reduces false negatives. Next-generation sequencing doubles the identification of pathogens in culture-negative TJA, often identifying polymicrobial infections previously overlooked [20]. Clarity reduces antibiotic guessing, initiating appropriate drugs 1 to 2 days earlier. Advanced imaging in positron emission tomography often spreads, directing debridement to precise locations. Point-of-care diagnostics identify 9 out of 10 infections bedside, accelerating decisions by 24 hours. These performance gains result in faster, better treatment of TJA patients.

Advances in treating total joint arthroplasty raise infection clearance and recovery of the patient to new heights in joint replacements. The 1.5-stage revision eradicates most of the infection, equal to a two-stage, yet the patient walks on crutches for weeks rather than months. VT-X7 pumps and phage therapy eradicate many resistant bugs, and some patients never need a second operation [21]. Silver-coated implants reduce infection in high-risk TJA without additional complications. Polymerase chain reaction, used during the operation, adjusts the course of treatment mid-case, increasing clearance in early adopters. These steps shorten the cycle of repeat procedures, providing a smoother ride back to normal for TJA patients.

Patient outcomes in total joint arthroplasty reflect the ripple effects of these advances in joint replacement. Rate of readmission due to postoperative infection have reduced in centers implementing new diagnostics and treatments, freeing beds, and alleviating costs. Pain subsides faster in the 1.5-stage or phage therapy patients by 3 months, compared to 6 months in traditional methods. Mobility is hastened, too—1.5-stage patients walk independently by 12 weeks, which is significantly faster than two-stage procedures, which usually takes months. Joint-function scores, such as the Harris Hip Score, increase with improved TJA management, reaching the 80s rather than the 70s as seen with traditional methods [21]. Quality-of-living questionnaires also show this, where anecdotal evidence shows patients with higher post-scores are more satisfied with their infection. These figures verify that technology raises the game in the TJA experience.

Prevention in total joint arthroplasty gains a technology boost, shaving infection rates before initiating joint replacement. Preoperative risk models identify many high-risk patients and initiate antibiotic cement or extended prophylaxis that reduces infection risk in certain groups. Photocatalyst coatings and silver implants reduce primary infection in pilot programs below regular metal implants. Intraoperative testing detects contamination in procedures, allowing surgeons to scrub it away prior to closure and saving many of those from becoming septic [22]. Predictive apps identify some additional early post-discharge infections, snuffing them out with outpatient medications. These layers reduce overall infection incidence in TJA, a significant consideration in a system that performs millions of procedures annually.

Challenges are still hanging over these advances in total joint arthroplasty, hindering their full impact on joint care. Costs are high with next-generation sequencing costing $1000 per pop, VT-X7 pumps costing $2000 per case, and silver implants adding thousands to bills for TJA. Many instruments lack large trials—phage therapy is based on 20 to 50-patient cohorts, hardly enough for gold-standard evidence. Training also comes slowly—molecular diagnostics requires lab techs, and AI requires data-aware surgeons, skills scarce in places besides big centers [23]. Rural TJA patients are the ones missing out, having to rely on old methods while city centers surge ahead, exacerbating outcome disparities. Adoption is slow until prices come down and evidence mounts.

Future potential in total joint arthroplasty shines brightly if these hurdles come down, portending even more significant gains for joint replacement. Phage therapy may strike mainstream TJA in terms of availability in 5 years, eradicating resistant infections for less than $500 per dose. Point-of-care tests may fall under $50, placing them in every clinic and detecting more infections. Artificial intelligence may complement the bright braces that monitor knee swelling alerting surgeons to infections pre-symptom [24]. Implant coatings may integrate silver, antibiotics, and phages, reducing primary TJA infections. These advances may change infection management, making TJA harder, faster, and fairer for all.

4. Conclusion

Total joint arthroplasty continues to shine as a vital solution in orthopedic surgery, restoring mobility and easing pain for countless patients through joint replacements. Infections remain a persistent barrier, threatening the benefits of this operation with their ability to derail recovery. Advances in technology in recent years have revolutionized how these infections are addressed, providing tools that support each level of care. Synovial biomarkers and molecular sequencing identify infections in TJA quickly and accurately compared to previous methods. Surgical procedures like the 1.5-stage revision and enhanced irrigation outcomes kill bacteria with greater efficacy, sparing patients additional surgeries. Phage therapy and antibiotic pumps kill resistant bacteria vigorously, increasing clearing capacity. New implants and risk models minimize infection risk before it happens. Patients experience the difference because pain disappears quicker, joints become functional earlier, and stays at the hospital are shorter. Surgeons use these technologies to protect the promise of total joint arthroplasty, minimizing previously intractable setbacks.

There are still challenges on the horizon for joint replacements, balancing the anticipation of these advances. Steep prices exclude technologies such as sequencing or coated implants from many budgets, particularly in smaller hospitals. Small early studies result in gaps in evidence, bringing caution to some surgeons' willingness to leap in. Training is a time-consuming proposition, and rural communities have few resources to keep pace, leading to uneven access across TJA care. These barriers challenge the field to meet higher expectations, proving that technology alone will not suffice without greater spread and bulletproof evidence. However, the future is promising. Affordable diagnostic tools may soon inundate clinics, causing infections the moment they occur in the operating room. Personalized treatments may wipe away resistant bacteria in sweeps. Real-time tracking may catch trouble in the moment, even before symptoms arise. Infection in total joint arthroplasty will never disappear. However, technology has turned the tide in favor of surgeons and their patients, paving the way for even more significant victories to come.

Author details

Varun Narula[1*], Sumit Anand[2], Ravindra Mohan[3] and Devang Bharti[4]

1 Department of Orthopedics, Delhi Cantonment General Hospital, Delhi, India

2 Department of Orthopedics, Miracles Apollo Spectra Hospital, Gurugram, Haryana, India

3 Department of Orthopedics, King George Medical College, Lucknow, India

4 Department of Anaesthesia, Lok Nayak Jai Prakash Narayan Hospital, Delhi, India

*Address all correspondence to: drvarunnarula1986@gmail.com

References

[1] Patel I, Nham F, Zalikha AK, El-Othmani MM. Epidemiology of total hip arthroplasty: Demographics, comorbidities, and outcomes. Arthroplasty. 2023;**5**:2. DOI: 10.1186/s42836-022-00156-1

[2] Rentschler S, Kaiser L, Deigner HP. Emerging options for the diagnosis of bacterial infections and the characterization of antimicrobial resistance. International Journal of Molecular Sciences. 2021;**22**:456. DOI: 10.3390/ijms22010456

[3] Xiao PL, Hsu CJ, Ma YG, Liu D, Peng R, Xu XH, et al. Prevalence and treatment rate of osteoporosis in patients undergoing total knee and hip arthroplasty: A systematic review and meta-analysis. Archives of Osteoporosis. 2022;**17**:16. DOI: 10.1007/s11657-021-01055-9

[4] Al-Jabri T, Ridha M, Wood MJ, Kayani B, Jayadev C, McCulloch RA, et al. An overview of the current diagnostic approach to periprosthetic joint infections. Orthopaedic Review. 2024;**16**:120308. DOI: 10.52965/001c.120308

[5] Sereda AP, Rukina AN, Trusova YV, Dzhavadov AA, Cherny AA, Bozhkova SA, et al. Dynamics of C-reactive protein level after orthopedic surgeries. Journal of Orthopaedics. 2024;**47**:1-7. DOI: 10.1016/j.jor.2023.11.014

[6] Palestro CJ. Molecular imaging of periprosthetic joint infections. Seminars in Nuclear Medicine. 2023;**53**:167-174. DOI: 10.1053/j.semnuclmed.2022.11.004

[7] Lai Y, Fan J, Lv N, Li X, Zhao W, Luo Z, et al. Neutrophil-lymphocyte ratio as predictor for acute infection after primary total joint arthroplasty in rheumatoid arthritis patients. Orthopaedic Surgery. May 2025;**17**(5):1314-1321. DOI: 10.1111/os.70002

[8] Pinski JM, Chen AF, Estok DM, Kavolus JJ. Nuclear medicine scans in total joint replacement. The Journal of Bone and Joint Surgery. American Volume. 2021;**103**:359-372. DOI: 10.2106/JBJS.20.00301

[9] Wang Z, Levin JE, Amen TB, Arzani A, Manzi JE, Lane JM. Total joint arthroplasty and osteoporosis: Looking beyond the joint to bone health. The Journal of Arthroplasty. 2022;**37**:1719-1725. DOI: 10.1016/j.arth.2022.04.010

[10] Russo A, Migliorini F, Giustra F, Bosco F, Massè A, Burastero G. Two-stage total joint replacement for hip or knee septic arthritis: Post-traumatic etiology and difficult-to-treat infections predict poor outcomes. Archives of Orthopaedic and Trauma Surgery. Dec 2024;**144**(12):5111-5119. DOI: 10.1007/s00402-024-05249-x

[11] Navarro G, Lozano L, Sastre S, Bori R, Bosch J, Bori G. Experiences during switching from two-stage to one-stage revision arthroplasty for chronic total knee arthroplasty infection. Antibiotics (Basel). 2021;**10**:1436. DOI: 10.3390/antibiotics10121436

[12] MacMahon A, Rao SS, Chaudhry YP, Hasan SA, Epstein JA, Hegde V, et al. Preoperative patient optimization in total joint arthroplasty—The paradigm shift from preoperative clearance: A narrative review. HSS Journal. 2022;**18**:418-427. DOI: 10.1177/15563316211030923

[13] Jevnikar BE, Ramos MS, Pasqualini I, Khan ST, Piuzzi NS. Effects of

elevated body mass index on total knee and hip arthroplasty success: A comprehensive overview. Expert Review of Medical Devices. 2025;**22**:75-87. DOI: 10.1080/17434440.2024.2444408

[14] Salem HS, Sherman AE, Chen Z, Scuderi GR, Mont MA. The utility of perioperative products for preventing surgical site infections in total knee arthroplasty and lower extremity arthroplasty: A systematic review. The Journal of Knee Surgery. 2022;**35**:1023-1043. DOI: 10.1055/s-0041-1740394

[15] Ricciardi BF, Muthukrishnan G, Masters EA, Kaplan N, Daiss JL, Schwarz EM. New developments and future challenges in the prevention, diagnosis, and treatment of prosthetic joint infection. Journal of Orthopaedic Research. 2020;**38**:1423-1435. DOI: 10.1002/jor.24595

[16] Indelli PF, Ghirardelli S, Violante B, Amanatullah DF. Next-generation sequencing for pathogen detection in periprosthetic joint infections. EFORT Open Reviews. 2021;**6**:236-244. DOI: 10.1302/2058-5241.6.200099

[17] Addissouky TA. Revolutionizing total knee arthroplasty: The integration and impact of artificial intelligence across the care continuum. Journal of Clinical Orthopaedics and Trauma Care. 2024;**6**:2694-0248. DOI: 10.31579/2694-0248/109

[18] Jevnikar BE, Khan ST, Huffman N, Pasqualini I, Surace PA, Deren ME, et al. Advancements in treatment strategies for periprosthetic joint infections: A comprehensive review. Journal of Clinical Orthopaedics and Trauma. 18 Jul 2024;**55**:102496. DOI: 10.1016/j.jcot.2024.102496

[19] Sequeira SB, Myntti MF, Lee J, Mont MA. An overview of research for the application of a novel biofilm-preventing surgical irrigation system for total joint arthroplasty procedures in order to reduce the risk of periprosthetic infection. Surgical Technology International. 2024;**44**:sti44-1780. DOI: 10.52198/24.STI.44.OS1780

[20] Feng JB, Chen R, Li B, Jiang BH, Li B. The current trend of antibacterial prostheses and prosthetic surface coating technologies to prevent prosthetic joint infection for artificial joint replacement. Journal of Biomaterials and Tissue Engineering. 2023;**13**:1046-1060. DOI: 10.1166/jbt.2023.3342

[21] Changjun C, Jingkun L, Yun Y, Yingguang W, Yanjun R, Debo Z, et al. Enhanced recovery after total joint arthroplasty (TJA): A contemporary systematic review of clinical outcomes and usage of key elements. Orthopaedic Surgery. 2023;**15**:1228-1240. DOI: 10.1111/os.13710

[22] Wang JC, Piple AS, Chen XT, Bedard NA, Callaghan JJ, Berry DJ, et al. The rise of medicare advantage: Effects on total joint arthroplasty patient care and research. The Journal of Bone and Joint Surgery. American Volume. 2022;**104**:2145-2152. DOI: 10.2106/JBJS.22.00254

[23] Martina K, Hunter DJ, Salmon LJ, Roe JP, Dowsey MM. Surgery for osteoarthritis: Total joint arthroplasty, realistic expectations of rehabilitation and surgical outcomes: A narrative review. Clinics in Geriatric Medicine. 2022;**38**:385-396. DOI: 10.1016/j.cger.2021.11.009

[24] Dubin JA, Bains SS, Hameed D, Gottlich C, Turpin R, Nace J, et al. Projected volume of primary total joint arthroplasty in the USA from 2019 to 2060. European Journal of Orthopaedic Surgery and Traumatology. 2024;**34**:2663-2670. DOI: 10.1007/s00590-024-03953-3

Chapter 4

Readmissions and Early Complications in Total Knee Arthroplasty Patients

Tushar Jethi, Deepak Jain, Rajnish Garg and Harpal Singh Selhi

Abstract

Total knee arthroplasty (TKA) improves pain, function, and quality of life, but rare complications can impact recovery. Identifying risk factors for complications and readmissions is crucial for better decision-making and patient outcomes. This study assessed readmission rates and early complications within 30 and 90 days after TKA. Out of 633 patients treated between January 2017 and February 2022, data from 609 were analyzed after excluding 28 due to unavailability. Hospital records were reviewed, and observations were recorded. The 30-day and 90-day readmission rates were 1.1% (n = 7) and 1.8% (n = 11), while unplanned visit rates were 2.6% (n = 16) at 30 days and 4.6% (n = 28) at 90 days. The 90-day unplanned readmission rate was 1.4% (n = 9), with causes categorized as medical (27.2%) and surgical (72.7%). No significant differences in readmissions or visits were found by age, body mass index (BMI), procedure type, or comorbidity status. Reoperation rates were 0.66% (n = 4) at 30 days and 1.15% (n = 8) at 90 days, with an average hospital stay of 6.53 days. The study concluded that readmission rates following TKA were low and were not significantly associated with patient factors like age, BMI, or comorbidities.

Keywords: total knee arthroplasty, length of stay, readmission, rates, causes, risk factors, prospective, retrospective, follow-up, reoperation

1. Introduction

The loss of articular cartilage, enlargement of bone at the borders, subchondral sclerosis, and a variety of biochemical and morphological changes to the synovial membrane and joint capsule are the hallmarks of knee osteoarthritis (OA), a chronic degenerative disease with a complex origin [1]. OA is hard to characterize, though, and its pathophysiology has to be better understood. A loss of cartilage linked to bone characteristics such as osteophytes and subchondral bone sclerosis is a common feature of all types of OA and related illnesses [2].

Age, sex, obesity, heredity, food, and joint damage are some of the risk factors for OA that differ from person to person based on the disease's stage [3]. Differentiating between single and clustered risk factors linked to the onset or progression of the disease is challenging.

The majority of treatments seek to enhance function and symptoms. Combining non-pharmacological, pharmaceutical, surgical, arthroscopic debridement, and lavage therapy methods is necessary for the best care of patients with knee OA [4]. In order to restore full function at the knee joint, significantly reduce pain, and improve function in patients with knee arthritis, total knee arthroplasty (TKA), sometimes referred to as "the gold standard," is a surgical procedure that replaces the articular surfaces of the knee joint (the tibial plateau and femoral condyles) with smooth metal and highly cross-linked polyethylene plastic [5]. When conservative therapy fails to alleviate OA symptoms in at least two of the knee's three compartments, total knee arthroscopy (TKA) is a popular and successful therapeutic option [6].

TKA is typically recommended for patients whose severe, chronic symptoms continue after all conservative and non-operative treatment alternatives have been exhausted. Patients with vascular dysfunction, neuroarthropathic degenerative joint disease, persistent remote (extra-articular) infection or bacteremia, or local knee infection (sepsis) should not have total knee arthroplasty [7].

Age, sex, and body mass index (BMI) are examples of demographic variables that have complex and varied effects. Different studies use different age intervals; some use a set number, while others use 5- or 10-year intervals. Increasing the age, weight, and physical activity of TKA patients may complicate matters, as may the way different studies classify predictive characteristics when evaluating risk [8].

Following total knee arthroplasty (TKA), the following complications can arise: pulmonary embolism, one of the most dreaded complications; deep vein thrombosis, one of the most dangerous and potentially fatal complications; infection, which is uncommon and only occurs in 2–3% of cases; and thromboembolism, one of the most serious complications. Following total knee arthroplasty (TKA), patellofemoral instability, extensor mechanism rupture, patellar fracture, patellar component failure, patellar component loosening, and patellar clunk syndrome are among the patellofemoral sequelae. Only 0.03% to 0.2% of patients experience neurovascular problems such as arterial damage following total knee arthroplasty (TKA), and 25% of these patients require amputation. After total knee arthroplasty, periprosthetic supracondylar femur fractures are also rare (0.3–2%) [9].

Readmission rates have gone up in tandem with the rise in the number of patients getting TKA. Finding the various avoidable reasons for readmission in TKA is made easier by researching the risk variables. Clinicians can gain a better understanding of their patients' postoperative course by knowing the risk factors for readmission after joint arthroplasty in a group of TKA recipients. The efficacy and efficiency of care will be enhanced by understanding potential risks, mitigation techniques, and how to identify patients who are most at risk of readmission [10].

Patients are most at risk of being readmitted to the hospital in the early post-surgical period, since the highest rates of hospital readmissions have been observed in the first 30 days following surgery. It is alarming that the post-TKA readmission rate for patients is between 5% and 8% [11]. Better post-surgical outcomes might have been achieved if patients had been better prepared for discharge following surgery and had a better understanding of the postoperative phase discharge instructions and guidelines, as evidenced by readmission [11].

More 30-day readmissions have been recorded as surgically related difficulties than readmissions from day 31 to day 90; specifically, 71% of the concerns during the first 30 days are related to surgery, compared to 47% of the remaining 60 days in a 90-day period. Ninety days is the ideal amount of time to report readmissions following joint replacement surgery [12]. Following TKA, there is a noticeable tendency toward shorter hospital stays (LOS). Additionally, the use of TKA surgery as an outpatient procedure has grown [13]. The ideal length of stay (LOS) after total knee arthroplasty (TKA) is still up for debate because LOS > 1 d after index surgery raises the likelihood of 90-d readmission, and a short LOS is linked to higher 30-d readmissionrates [14].

The Indian people have a dearth of books on this subject. In order to investigate complications and risk factors in this patient population, the current study was carried out to examine the readmission pattern among patients who had primary total knee arthroplasty.

2. Risk factors for complications following total knee arthroplasty

Total Knee Arthroplasty (TKA) is generally associated with favorable outcomes, but a proportion of patients experience complications that lead to unplanned hospital visits or readmissions. Several factors influence the likelihood of these complications, including patient demographics, comorbidities, and hospital factors. This section explores the risk factors identified in our study, compares them with existing literature, and discusses the implications for clinical practice.

2.1 Age

Age is a well-recognized factor influencing the risk of complications following TKA. In our cohort, the mean age of patients was 62.87 years, with no significant correlation between age and the likelihood of unplanned visits or readmissions within 90 days postoperatively ($p = 0.922$). This is consistent with findings from Schairer et al. [15] and Gromov et al. [16], where no significant age differences were observed between readmitted and non-readmitted patients. However, other studies, such as those by Ali et al. [17] and D'Apuzzo et al. [18], have shown that older age groups (>65 or >75 years) are at a higher risk for readmissions, particularly when comorbidities are present. Furthermore, studies like those by Yohe et al. [19] have highlighted that patients aged over 84 years' experience an increased risk of minor complications.

2.2 Sex

In our study, 69% of the enrolled patients were female, a common trend observed in TKA patient populations. Interestingly, despite the higher female representation, our data revealed that male patients had significantly higher comorbidities ($p = 0.003$). These findings align with those of Urish et al. [20] and Gould et al. [8], who found that male sex was associated with an increased risk of readmission. However, contradictory findings were reported by Schairer et al. [15] and Yohe et al. [19], where no significant relationship between sex and readmission rates was observed.

2.3 Comorbidities

The presence of comorbid conditions is a significant predictor of postoperative complications following TKA. In our study, hypertension was the most common comorbidity, affecting 32.8% of patients, followed by diabetes (14.4%) and coronary artery disease (4.4%). We found a correlation between high comorbidity scores and prolonged length of stay ($p = 0.001$), as well as a longer duration of knee pain prior to surgery. Although high comorbidity status did not correlate with increased unplanned visits or readmissions within 30 and 90 days ($p > 0.05$), it is consistent with findings by Benito et al. [14], who reported diabetes and coronary artery disease as predictors of 90-day readmission. Other studies, such as those by Fischer et al. [21] and D'Apuzzo et al. [18], also support that conditions like diabetes, hypertension, and coagulopathy are significant risk factors for readmission following TKA.

2.4 Body mass index (BMI)

In our study, 54.5% of patients had a BMI greater than 25, indicating overweight status. A higher BMI has been shown to correlate with a higher incidence of comorbidities, and in our analysis, patients with higher BMI had more significant comorbidity profiles ($p = 0.001$). Several studies have found that obesity, along with related conditions like diabetes and hypertension, is associated with higher complication rates and increased risk of readmission [18, 22]. Although our study did not show a direct correlation between BMI and unplanned readmissions ($p = 0.633$), other literature suggests that patients with a BMI >30 are at higher risk of infection and wound complications post-TKA [15, 19].

2.5 Length of hospital stay (LOS)

In our study, the mean length of stay (LOS) post-TKA was found to be relatively short, consistent with the global trend toward shorter hospital stays for TKA patients. This reduction in LOS, however, has been linked to higher readmission rates in other studies [14]. Urish et al. [20] found that patients with longer LOS, particularly those older and diabetic, had an increased risk of reoperation within one year. However, in our study, patients who had a longer LOS did not demonstrate a significant increase in unplanned readmissions, possibly due to the comprehensive pre-discharge optimization strategies in place.

2.6 Surgical and wound complications

Surgical complications, particularly wound-related issues, were among the most common causes of unplanned hospital visits in our cohort. Five patients developed surgical site wound complications at the 30-day follow-up, with four requiring readmission. Wound infection and surgical complications remain one of the most common reasons for readmission in TKA patients, as observed in studies by Schairer et al. [15] and D'Apuzzo et al. [18]. In our study, 11% of readmissions within the 90-day period were due to surgical causes, including infection and soft tissue injuries, which is consistent with findings from Schairer et al. [15], who found that surgical complications accounted for three-fourths of readmissions.

2.7 Unplanned readmissions

Our study reported an overall unplanned readmission rate of 1.1% within 30 days and 1.8% within 90 days. This rate is lower compared to studies like those by Urish et al. [20], who reported a 4% readmission rate within 30 days. This may reflect differences in healthcare systems, patient optimization, or post-discharge care. Notably, our study found that most unplanned readmissions were due to surgical complications (four of seven readmissions within 30 days), aligning with global data indicating that infection and wound complications are the leading causes of readmission after TKA.

DOI: http://dx.doi.org/10.5772/intechopen.1010101

3. Global trends in readmission after total knee arthroplasty (TKA)

Total knee arthroplasty (TKA) has become a common procedure for managing advanced knee arthritis and improving patients' quality of life. However, unplanned readmissions following TKA present significant challenges, impacting healthcare costs, patient satisfaction, and clinical outcomes. This section explores global trends, risk factors, and preventive strategies for readmissions after TKA based on data from various studies conducted worldwide.

3.1 Readmission rates and common causes

Studies have revealed considerable variation in 30-day readmission rates after TKA across regions and healthcare systems:

- Apuzzo et al. (USA) found a 30-day readmission rate of 5.8% in a cohort of 377,705 patients. Gastrointestinal bleeding and periprosthetic infections were significant causes [18].

- Workman et al. (USA) reported a readmission rate of 2.8% among 7482 patients, with gastrointestinal bleeding (9.05%) and periprosthetic infection (8.10%) being the most common reasons [23].

- Avram et al. (Canada) observed a 5.3% readmission rate, with surgical site infections (23.2%) and cardiovascular events (16.8%) being the leading causes [24].

3.2 Risk factors for readmission

3.2.1 Patient-related risk factors

- Comorbidities: Gould et al. [8] highlighted the influence of conditions such as diabetes, chronic kidney disease (CKD), cardiovascular disease, and bleeding disorders on readmissions.

- Age and BMI: Yohe et al. [19] found that elderly patients (especially those over 84 years) and individuals with a high body mass index (BMI) had increased readmission rates.

- Socioeconomic status: Ali et al. [17] identified lower socioeconomic status as a predictor of all-cause and surgical readmissions.

3.2.2 Procedural factors

- Length of stay (LOS): Benito et al. [14] demonstrated that a longer LOS beyond one day was associated with higher 90-day readmissions.

- Same-day discharge: Gromov et al. [16] found no significant safety concerns associated with same-day discharge when strict selection criteria were applied.

- Surgical techniques: Ali et al. [17] reported a lower risk of readmission with unicompartmental arthroplasty compared to total knee arthroplasty.

3.2.3 Systemic and healthcare-related factors

- Hospital volume: Apuzzo et al. [18] noted an association between higher hospital volumes and lower readmission rates.

- Institutional practices: Piuzzi et al. [25] emphasized the role of hospital site and surgeon-related factors in predicting LOS and readmission risk.

3.3 Temporal trends in readmission and mortality

Berstock et al. [26] observed a global decline in 30- and 90-day mortality rates following TKA over the past two decades, potentially due to improvements in perioperative care and patient selection [13, 27].

3.4 Methodological considerations

Fischer et al. [21] conducted a systematic review to assess the validity of readmission rates as a quality indicator for hospital care. They highlighted challenges related to case-mix correction, competing outcomes, and data reliability.

3.5 Prevention strategies and future directions

3.5.1 Identifying high-risk patients

Predictive models incorporating demographic and clinical factors, such as those proposed by Gould et al. [8, 28], can help identify patients at higher risk of readmission. These models consider variables such as patient age, comorbidities, and previous surgical history to assess the likelihood of complications and unplanned hospital returns.

3.5.2 Optimizing perioperative care

Efforts should focus on improving discharge planning and post-discharge monitoring. Gould et al. [8] suggested closer monitoring during the early post-discharge period to reduce avoidable readmissions. Strategies include enhanced recovery protocols, better coordination between inpatient and outpatient care, and early identification of potential postoperative complications.

3.5.3 Addressing comorbidities

Proper management of chronic conditions is critical to reducing readmission risks. Gould et al. [8] and Yohe et al. [19] emphasized the importance of managing cardiovascular disease, chronic kidney disease (CKD), and diabetes in patients undergoing total knee arthroplasty (TKA). Optimizing these conditions prior to surgery and maintaining adequate control postoperatively can significantly decrease complications.

3.5.4 Enhancing patient education and support

Improving patient education and support systems plays a key role in reducing readmissions. Saucedo et al. [29] recommended comprehensive education programs that emphasize lifestyle interventions, medication compliance, and postoperative care instructions. By empowering patients with knowledge and resources, healthcare providers can improve adherence to care protocols and reduce the likelihood of complications.

The global trends in readmission after TKA underscore the need for a multi-faceted approach involving patient selection, surgical techniques, perioperative care, and post-discharge monitoring. By addressing key risk factors and adopting evidence-based practices, healthcare providers can improve outcomes, reduce readmissions, and enhance the overall effectiveness of TKA procedures (**Figures 1–3** and **Tables 1–6**).

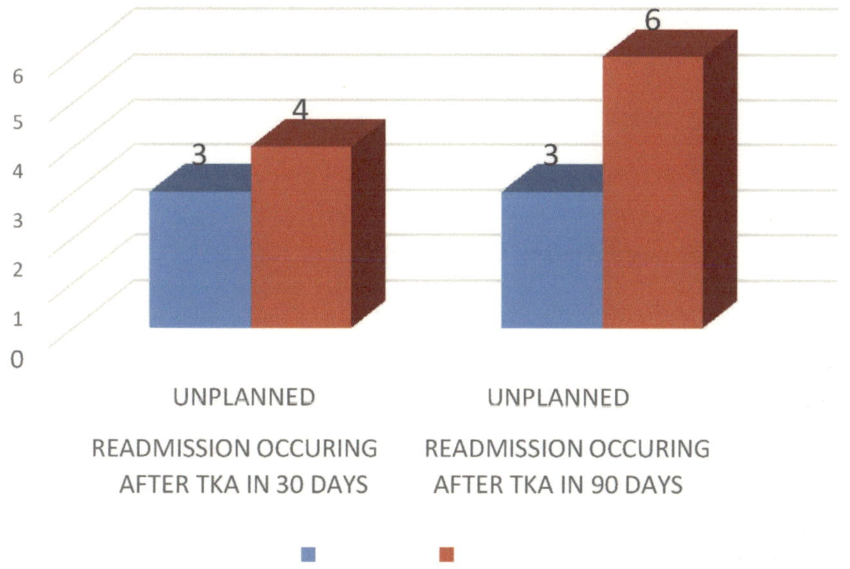

Figure 1.
Distribution of patients according to reasons for readmissions at 30 days and 90 days follow-up after TKA.

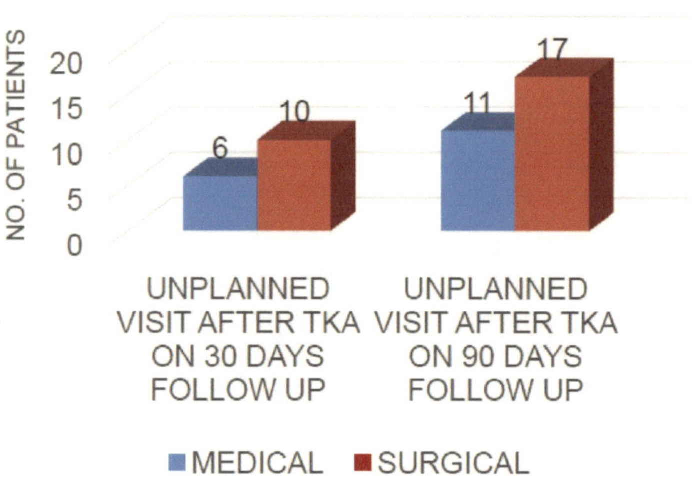

Figure 2.
Distribution of patients according to reasons for unplanned visits at 30 days and 90 days follow-up after TKA.

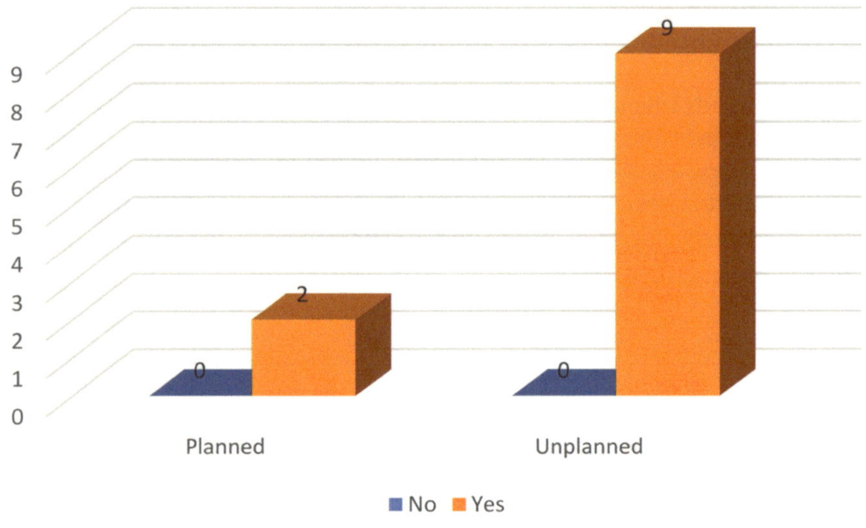

Figure 3.
Table for unplanned and planned readmissions within 90 days.

Study variable		Cases, *n*	Percent
Age in year	≤ 40	5	0.8
	41–50	43	7.1
	51–60	197	32.3
	61–70	251	41.2
	71–80	104	17.1
	> 80	9	1.5
Sex	Female	420	69
	Male	189	31
Body mass index in kg/m^2	< 24.9 (normal)	249	40.8
	25–29.9 (overweight)	332	54.5
	> 30 (class 1 obesity)	28	4.6
Diagnosis	Osteoarthritis	593	97.4
	Rheumatoid arthritis	16	2.6
Laterality	Bilateral	304	49.9
	Unilateral	305	50.1
Duration of complaint	< 1	3	0.5
	1–2.0	26	4.3
	2–5.0	168	27.6
	5–10.0	239	39.2
	> 10	173	28.4

DOI: http://dx.doi.org/10.5772/intechopen.1010101

Study variable		Cases, *n*	Percent
Charlson comorbidity index	< 2	399	65.5
	2–3.0	156	25.6
	> 4	54	8.9
Length of stay in d	6	297	48.8
	7	306	50.2
	8	4	0.7
	10	1	0.2
	13	1	0.2

Table 1.
Characteristics of the study population.

Unplanned visit after TKA within 30 d	Follow-up	Cases, *n*	Percent
Occurred?	No	593	97.40
	Yes	16	2.60
Reason	Febrile illness	2	0.40
	Urinary tract infection	2	0.40
	Neurological issues	1	0.20
	Lower back ache	1	0.20
	Post-TKA pain	3	0.60
	Wound complications	5	1.00
	Other surgery-related complications	2	0.40

TKA: Total knee arthroplasty.

Table 2.
Unplanned visits within 30 d after total knee arthroplasty.

Unplanned visit after TKA within 30 d	Follow-up	Cases, *n*	Percent
Occurred?	No	815	95.40
	Yes	8	4.60
Reason for unplanned visits within 90 d	Febrile illness	3	0.60
	Urinary tract infection	3	0.60
	Neurological issues	2	0.40
	Generalized body weakness	1	0.20
	Lower back ache	2	0.40
	Soft tissue injury over knee	2	0.40
	Post-TKA pain	7	1.40
	Wound complications	5	1.00
	Other surgery-related complication	3	0.60

TKA: Total knee arthroplasty.

Table 3.
Unplanned visits within 90 d after total knee arthroplasty.

Reasons for readmissions within 90 d	Cases, *n*	Percent
Febrile illness	2	0.40
Neurological issues	2	0.40
Talonavicular degeneration	1	0.20
Soft tissue injury over knee	2	0.40
Wound complications	4	0.80

Table 4.
Reasons for readmissions at 90 d.

Readmission after TKA	On 30-d follow-up	On 90-d follow-up
Our study	1.1% (n = 7)	1.8% (n = 11)
Urish *et al.* [20]	4% (n = 703)	5.8% (n = 1209)
Cassard *et al.* [30]	3.3% (n = 2) outpatient 4.9% (n = 25) inpatient	NA
Avram *et al.* [24]	2% (n = 55)	NA
Workman *et al.* [23]	2.8% (n = 210)	NA
Ali *et al.* [17]	6.0% (n = 37,195)	NA
Apuzzo *et al.* [18]	5.8% (n = 22,076)	NA

NA: Not available; TKA: Total knee arthroplasty.

Table 5.
Comparisons of readmissions after total knee arthroplasty in various studies.

Unplanned readmission after TKA	On 30-d follow-up	On 90-d follow-up
In our study	1.1% (n = 7)	1.4% (n = 9)
Schairer *et al.* [15]	4% (n = 57)	8% (n = 118)
Urish *et al.* [20]	4% (n = 703)	5.8% (n = 1209)
Cassard *et al.* [30]	3.3% (n = 2) outpatient 4.9% (n = 25) inpatient	NA
Apuzzo *et al.* [18]	5.8% (n = 22,076)	NA
Springer *et al.* [31]	12% outpatient* 6% inpatient*	NA
Ali *et al.* [17]	6.0% (n = 37,195)	NA
Workman *et al.* [23]	2.8% (n = 210)	NA
Avram *et al.* [24]	2% (n = 55)	NA
Yohe *et al.* [19]	4.7% (n = 566)	NA

**Number data not reported. NA: Not available; TKA: Total knee arthroplasty.*

Table 6.
Comparisons of unplanned readmissions after total knee arthroplasty in various studies.

4. Conclusions

In conclusion, while age, sex, and comorbidities are frequently cited risk factors for complications following TKA, our study found that none of these factors were strongly correlated with unplanned readmissions or visits within 90 days postoperatively. Surgical complications, particularly wound issues, were the primary causes of unplanned readmissions. This highlights the importance of stringent perioperative care, appropriate patient optimization, and early intervention for surgical complications to minimize the risk of readmission and improve patient outcomes. Further research with larger sample sizes and varied populations is necessary to validate these findings, especially in settings like India, where healthcare infrastructure and practices may differ.

Acknowledgements

The author would like to express their gratitude to Dr. Deepak Jain (Professor, Department of Orthopedics, DMC&H, Ludhiana) for mentoring guidance and Dr. Rajnish Garg (Professor and Head, Department of Orthopedics, DMC&H, Ludhiana) for additional scholarly guidance in the completion of this study.

Conflict of interest

The authors declare no conflict of interest.

Abbreviations

ASA	American society of anesthesiologists
DVT	deep vein thrombosis
DOS	day of surgery
ESR	erythrocyte sedimentation rate
LOS	length of stay
LMWH	low molecular weight heparin
IL	interleukin
MRI	magnetic resonance imaging
NSAIDS	non-steroidal anti-inflammatory drugs
OA	osteoarthritis
ORIF	open reduction and internal fixation
PFA	patello femoral arthritis
PE	pulmonary Embolism
PRBC	packed red blood cell
PRE-OP	pre-operatively
POST-OP	post operatively
RTT	return to theater
RA	rheumatoid Arthritis
RNA	ribonucleic acid

TNF	*tumor necrosis factor*
THA	total hip arthroplasty
TKA	total knee arthroplasty
TJA	total joint arthroplasty
UTI	urinary tract infection
VAC	vacuum assisted closure

Author details

Tushar Jethi*, Deepak Jain, Rajnish Garg and Harpal Singh Selhi
Department of Orthopedic Surgery, Dayanand Medical College and Hospital, Ludhiana, Punjab, India

*Address all correspondence to: tj.saiyaman@gmail.com

References

[1] Firestein GS, Budd RC, Gabriel SE, McInnes IB, O'Dell JR. Etiology and pathogenesis of rheumatoid arthritis. In: Koretzky G, editor. Kelly's Textbook of Rheumatology. 2009. pp. 1035-1086. DOI: 10.1016/B978-1-4160-3285-4.10065-8

[2] Courtney PM, Rozell JC, Melnic CM, Lee GC. Who should not undergo short stay hip and knee arthroplasty? Risk factors associated with major medical complications following primary total joint arthroplasty. The Journal of Arthroplasty. 2015;**30**(1):1-4. DOI: 10.1016/j.arth.2015.01.056

[3] Abramoff B, Caldera FE. Osteoarthritis: Pathology, diagnosis, and treatment options. The Medical Clinics of North America. 2020;**104**(2):293-311. DOI: 10.1016/j.mcna.2019.10.007

[4] Gross DE, Brenner SL, Esformes I, Gross ML. Arthroscopic treatment of degenerative joint disease of the knee. Orthopedics. 1991;**14**(12):1317-1321. DOI: 10.3928/0147-7447-19911201-06

[5] Robertsson O, Knutson K, Lewold S, Lidgren L. The Swedish knee arthroplasty register 1975-1997: An update with special emphasis on 41,223 knees operated on in 1988-1997. Acta Orthopaedica Scandinavica. 2001;**72**(6):503-513. DOI: 10.1080/000164701753532853

[6] Hsu H, Siwiec RM. Knee arthroplasty. In: StatPearls [Internet]. Treasure Island (FL): StatPearls Publishing; 2024. p. 2023 [cited 2023]

[7] Varacallo M, Luo TD, Johanson NA. Total knee arthroplasty techniques. In: StatPearls [Internet]. Treasure Island (FL): StatPearls Publishing; 2024. Available from: https://www.ncbi.nlm.nih.gov/books/NBK499896/ [Accessed: 4 August 2023]

[8] Gould D, Dowsey MM, Spelman T, Jo O, Kabir W, Trieu J, et al. Patient-related risk factors for unplanned 30-day hospital readmission following primary and revision total knee arthroplasty: A systematic review and meta-analysis. Journal of Clinical Medicine. 2021;**10**(1):134. DOI: 10.3390/jcm10010134

[9] Courtney PM, Boniello AJ, Berger RA. Complications following outpatient total joint arthroplasty: An analysis of a national database. The Journal of Arthroplasty. 2017;**32**(5):1426-1430. DOI: 10.1016/j.arth.2016.11.055

[10] Zuckerman RB, Sheingold SH, Orav EJ, Ruhter J, Epstein AM. Readmissions, observation, and the hospital readmissions reduction program. The New England Journal of Medicine. 2016;**374**(16):1543-1551. DOI: 10.1056/NEJMsa1513024

[11] Pamilo KJ, Torkki P, Peltola M, Pesola M, Remes V, Paloneva J. Fast-tracking for total knee replacement reduces use of institutional care without compromising quality. Acta Orthopaedica. 2018;**89**(2):184-189. DOI: 10.1080/17453674.2017.1399643

[12] Kurtz SM, Lau EC, Ong KL, Adler EM, Kolisek FR, Manley MT. Which hospital and clinical factors drive 30- and 90-day readmission after TKA? The Journal of Arthroplasty. 2016;**31**(10):2099-2107. DOI: 10.1016/j.arth.2016.03.045

[13] Bozic KJ, Chiu V. Emerging ideas: Shared decision making in patients

with osteoarthritis of the hip and knee. Clinical Orthopaedics and Related Research. 2011;**469**(7):2081-2085. DOI: 10.1007/s11999-010-1740-7

[14] Benito J, Stafford J, Judd H, Ng M, Corces A, Roche MW. Length of stay increases 90-day readmission rates in patients undergoing primary total joint arthroplasty. JAAOS Global Research and Reviews. 2022;**6**(3):e21.00271. DOI: 10.5435/JAAOSGlobal-D-21-00271

[15] Schairer WW, Vail TP, Bozic KJ. What are the rates and causes of hospital readmission after total knee arthroplasty? Clinical Orthopaedics and Related Research. 2014;**472**(1):181-187. DOI: 10.1007/s11999-013-3030-7

[16] Schmidt AM, Garval M, Gromov K, Holm C, Larsen JR, Runge C, et al. Feasibility, safety, and patient-reported outcomes 90 days after same-day total knee arthroplasty: A matched cohort study. Acta Orthopaedica. 2022;**93**(5):509-518. DOI: 10.2340/17453674.2022.2807

[17] Ali AM, Bottle A. The validity of all-cause 30-day readmission rate as a hospital performance metric after primary total hip and knee arthroplasty: A systematic review. The Journal of Arthroplasty. 2019;**34**(8):1831-1836. DOI: 10.1016/j.arth.2019.04.011

[18] D'Apuzzo M, Westrich G, Hidaka C, Pan TJ, Lyman S. All-cause versus complication-specific readmission following total knee arthroplasty. The Journal of Bone and Joint Surgery. American Volume. 2017;**99**(13):1093. DOI: 10.2106/JBJS.16.00874

[19] Yohe N, Funk A, Ciminero M, Erez O, Saleh A. Complications and readmissions after total knee replacement in octogenarians and nonagenarians. Geriatric Orthopaedic Surgery and Rehabilitation. 2018;**9**:2151459318804113. DOI: 10.1177/2151459318804113

[20] Urish KL, Qin Y, Li BY, Borza T, Sessine M, Kirk P, et al. Predictors and cost of readmission in total knee arthroplasty. The Journal of Arthroplasty. 2018;**33**(9):2759-2763. DOI: 10.1016/j.arth.2018.04.008

[21] Fischer C, Lingsma HF, Marang-van de Mheen PJ, Kringos DS, Klazinga NS, et al. Is the readmission rate a valid quality indicator? A review of the evidence. PLoS One. 2014;**9**:e112282. DOI: 10.1371/journal.pone.0112282

[22] Li BY, Urish KL, Jacobs BL, He C, Borza T, Qin Y, et al. Inaugural readmission penalties for total hip and total knee arthroplasty procedures under the hospital readmissions reduction program. JAMA Network Open. 2019;**2**:e1916008

[23] Workman KK, Angerett N, Lippe R, Shin A, King S. Thirty-day unplanned readmission after total knee arthroplasty at a teaching community hospital: Rates, reasons, and risk factors. The Journal of Knee Surgery. 2020;**33**:206-212. DOI: 10.1055/s-0038-1677510

[24] Avram V, Petruccelli D, Winemaker M, de Beer J. Total joint arthroplasty readmission rates and reasons for 30-day hospital readmission. The Journal of Arthroplasty. 2014;**29**(3):465-468. DOI: 10.1016/j.arth.2013.07.039

[25] Piuzzi N, Strnad G, Esa W, Barsoum W, Bloomfield M, Brooks P, et al. The main predictors of length of stay after total knee arthroplasty: Patient-related or procedure-related risk factors. JBJS. 2019;**101**:1093-1101. DOI: 10.2106/JBJS.18.00758

[26] Berstock JR, Beswick AD, Lopez-Lopez JA, et al. Mortality after total

knee arthroplasty: A systematic review of incidence, temporal trends, and risk factors. JBJS. 2018;**100**(12):e49. DOI: 10.2106/JBJS.17.00249

[27] Cram P, Lu X, Kates SL, Singh JA, Li Y, Wolf BR. Total knee arthroplasty volume, utilization, and outcomes among Medicare beneficiaries, 1991-2010. Journal of the American Medical Association. 2012;**308**:1227-1236. DOI: 10.1001/2012.jama.11153

[28] Gould D, Dowsey M, Spelman T, Jo I, Kabir W, Trieu J, et al. Patient-related risk factors for unplanned 30-day readmission following total knee arthroplasty: A protocol for a systematic review and meta-analysis. Systematic Reviews. 2019;**8**(1):1-8. DOI: 10.1186/s13643-019-1140-3

[29] Saucedo JM, Marecek GS, Wanke TR, Lee J, Stulberg SD, Puri L. Understanding readmission after primary total hip and knee arthroplasty: Who's at risk? The Journal of Arthroplasty. 2014;**29**(2):256-260

[30] Cassard X, Garnault V, Corin B, Claverie D, Murgier J. Outpatient total knee arthroplasty: Readmission and complication rates on day 30 in 61 patients. Orthopaedics & Traumatology, Surgery & Research. 2018;**104**(7):967-970. DOI: 10.1016/j.otsr.2018.07.014

[31] Odum SM, Springer BD. In-hospital complication rates and associated factors after simultaneous bilateral vs unilateral total knee arthroplasty. JBJS. 2014;**96**:1058-1065. DOI: 10.2106/JBJS.M.00065

Chapter 5

Extended Trochanteric Osteotomy

James Toale, Mohamed Ahmed and James M. Broderick

Abstract

Extended trochanteric osteotomy (ETO) is a valuable technique in revision total hip arthroplasty, facilitating enhanced exposure to the femoral canal and acetabulum, particularly in cases with well-fixed implants, significant femoral deformity or severe osteolysis. Understanding of this technique is essential for arthroplasty surgeons. This technique aids in component removal while preserving surrounding structures. Since its initial description ETO has evolved, with modifications in technique, indications and fixation strategies. This chapter will provide a comprehensive overview of ETO, including its indications, techniques, variations, technical considerations and various osteotomy fixation methods. Additionally, it will discuss outcomes, complications, and post-operative protocols, incorporating the latest evidence. By understanding these principles, surgeons can optimise patient outcomes and minimise complications associated with complex revision hip surgery.

Keywords: extended trochanteric osteotomy, revision, hip arthroplasty, exposure, hip replacement

1. Introduction

Extended trochanteric osteotomy (ETO) is a powerful and versatile tool that is an essential skill for modern arthroplasty surgeons, particularly those who perform revision total hip arthroplasty. Multiple prior techniques to access the femoral shaft have been described in the past, which have aimed to improve exposure and aid implant removal in particular. Notably, Sir John Charnley described a transtrochanteric approach for use in both primary and revision surgeries, and this formed the basis of both primary and revision total hip arthroplasty for many years. Further techniques, all with the aim of improving femoral access, particularly in the revision setting, were described including trochanteric slide osteotomies and transfemoral osteotomies. While these techniques maintain relevance in certain settings, the extended trochanteric osteotomy has gained popularity in recent times due to its versatility, utility and favourable outcome profile.

Younger et al. popularised the extended trochanteric osteotomy technique, which involves an osteotomy of the greater trochanter and various lengths of the femoral diaphysis in order to gain access to the medullary canal. In principle, the osteotomised bone, which is levered anteriorly, maintains its muscle attachments. Gluteus medius and minimus attachments as well as the origin of vastus lateralis (with periosteal attachments) aid in maintaining blood supply to bone fragments for healing and prevent proximal bone fragment translation, which was a complication seen with previous osteotomy techniques. While its utility has broadened over time, its technique has been refined with the goal of optimising outcomes. This chapter will explore ETO and provide updates with the latest evidence to support it.

2. Techniques

Initially described by Wagner et al. and later popularised by Younger et al., they described the ETO technique using the anterolateral approach in 1995 [1, 2]. This is a largely anteriorly based technique compared to the laterally based Paprosky method. Following a standard anterolateral (or lateral) approach and exposure of the posterior proximal femur, the vastus lateralis is dissected off the femur while maintaining its attachment at the vastus ridge. The osteotomy is then marked just anterolateral to the linea aspera, extending from the quadrate tubercle of the greater trochanter to a predetermined distal point. A high-speed burr (or oscillating saw) is then used to perforate the posterior cortex and extend to the anterolateral cortex at various points along the marked line. The burr holes are then connected using a saw or osteotome on the posterior cortex. The distal lateral cut is also performed using an oscillating saw. Lambotte osteotomes are then passed through the posterior osteotomy to pierce the anterolateral cortex. They are then levered to lift the osteotomy fragment anteriorly in a controlled manner. The osteotomy should involve the posterior one-third of the femur only. This method leaves the attachments of gluteus medius, gluteus minimus and vastus lateralis intact.

In comparison, Paprosky et al. (2003) describe a similar technique with some differences. It involves an approach to the lateral cortex (Wagner et al. lift the anterior cortex), which they describe through the posterior approach to the hip. Using a saw, the posterolateral one-third of the proximal femur is osteotomised. In their description, they describe the use of an oscillating saw to perforate both the posterior and anterior cortices and the use of a pencil reamer for the distal/lateral cut. In their series of 122 patients, they described excellent results including high union rates and quicker operative times [3]. Similar methods were described by Chen et al. who performed the anterior cut from distal to proximal using an oscillating saw distally followed by a 1.3 cm osteotome. The osteotomy site was bevelled in their series [4].

Lakstein et al. (2011) describe their technique which aims to maintain the posterior hip capsule and short external rotators to improve hip stability [5]. This method involves approaching the hip through the lateral approach. The posterior osteotomy is made initially, extending from the tip of the greater trochanter. The cut is made posterior to the gluteus medius insertion and anterior to the insertion site of the short external rotators. The cut is extended distally to involve the lateral one-third of the femur diaphysis. The osteotomy is levered anteriorly, maintaining the attachments of the gluteus minimus, gluteus medius and vastus lateralis while maintaining the short external rotator attachments posteriorly.

In recent years, the popularity of the direct anterior approach for hip arthroplasty has increased, particularly in the primary setting. One of the concerns regarding the direct anterior approach was its suitability for revision surgery and the potential difficulty in the removal of a well-fixed femoral stem. These concerns largely stem from the difficulty of extending the approach distally for improved visualisation. Compared to the posterior approach, for example, distal extension is less accessible, making ETO more difficult. Distal exposure techniques include vastus lateralis split and a posterior-directed S-shaped incision. That said, Morcos et al. (2020) described a technique for

ETO following the direct anterior approach. Following the approach and adequate exposure distally, an oscillating saw is used to cut from the anterolateral femur to the posterior cortex. The cut is extended laterally at the distal aspect. Using osteotomes, the osteotomy fragment is displaced laterally to expose the canal [6]. For now, posterior, direct lateral and anterolateral approaches remain the work-horse approaches for revision surgery and, as such, for the performance of ETO, although as the direct anterior approach is popularised, so too may its use in revision surgery be improved.

In terms of planning and accuracy, it has been suggested in cadaveric studies that the use of 3D cutting guides could allow for a more accurate and patient-specific osteotomy, which could prevent iatrogenic fracture and soft tissue injury, although it has not become the norm yet [7].

There have been previous concerns about the use of cemented implants following ETO due to the theoretical risk of cement leakage into the fracture site and thermal necrosis of osteoblasts, both potentially preventing or delaying healing. Evidence has shown that cement can be safely used in revision surgery after ETO [8, 9]. It is advised that particular care is taken to fixation of the fragment. There should be anatomical reduction without gapping and adequate fixation to counteract the cement pressurisation phase and to prevent cement extrusion, which may lead to delayed or non-union.

Modifications of techniques continue to evolve. Examples where modifications are necessary are in the setting of a periprosthetic fracture for revision stem, for example, where incorporation of the fracture line into the ETO may be necessary. Overall, it is sensible to choose an approach that is suitable to the approach performed. For example, the Paprosky approach is more easily performed following a posterior approach to the proximal femur. It is important that the technique most appropriate to the approach being performed and the individual patient setting is planned for and performed. Whatever approach is used, the principles should be adhered to with regard to maintaining soft tissue attachments in particular.

3. Indications/patient selection

ETO is primarily utilised in the revision hip arthroplasty setting, although its indications and utility continue to expand. It is often planned pre-operatively, although commonly, an intra-operative decision is made to utilise the approach when conventional methods have failed or when the risk of iatrogenic injury is considered higher than the risk of ETO.

3.1 Removal of femoral implants

The majority of revision cases are in the setting of aseptic loosening and therefore the majority of ETO's are used in cases of aseptic loosening. Controlled extraction of implants by direct medullary visualisation can reduce intra-operative fracture rates and complications.

ETO is utilised in the removal of both cemented and uncemented implants. In cemented implants, an effective ETO can give exposure to the full cement mantle to the distal tip centraliser, allowing for the successful removal of the entire cement mantle without unwanted cortical perforation. Pre-planning with accurate templating allows for cut length measurements that will allow for sufficient exposure while minimising unnecessary osteotomy distal extension. Minimising unwanted distal extension allows for optimal length of distal stem fixation, which will provide optimum implant stability. Multiple studies have described ETO for well-fixed cemented implant removal with successful results [10, 11]. ETO allows for direct vision of the cement mantle within the canal and certainty that the entire cement mantle is removed. If a revision is required with an uncemented stem, it is important that the entire cement mantle is removed to expose underlying cortical bone for optimum femoral component osteointegration. Through direct visualisation of the femoral canal, the removal of cement is easier and more accurate. Direct visualisation of the canal also allows for easier irrigation of canal-infected cases. Well-fixed uncemented stems occasionally require ETO for extraction following the failure of conventional methods. The approach is similar to that of cemented implants but without the requirement for cement removal.

3.2 Acetabulum exposure or removal of acetabular implants

Although only occasionally used as its primary indication, ETO can be used to improve acetabular exposure. ETO can allow for improved femoral mobilisation and retraction, which can aid in acetabular exposure. In cases such as high-riding greater trochanter (dysplasia), post-traumatic deformities, proximal femoral stiffness and excessive greater trochanter bone overgrowth, ETO can allow for improved acetabular exposure prior to femoral preparation. This exposure can be utilised for both acetabular preparation and removal of acetabular implants. Some have described the successful use of ETO in the removal of acetabular components that have become displaced to an intra-pelvic position [12].

3.3 Periprosthetic hip infection

ETO can be used in the setting of periprosthetic hip infection, particularly in the setting of two-stage revision surgery for the removal of primary implants and improved exposure. Concerns regarding the use of ETO in the setting of infection lie with the potentially higher risk for ETO non-union and the requirement for further metalwork for ETO fixation that may harbour infection and prevent adequate infection eradication. Advocates for its use in a two-stage revision would argue that ETO allows for safe femoral component extraction, complete removal of cement and thorough irrigation of the canal under direct visualisation with debridement. Evidence has shown that both immediate and delayed ETO fixation (leaving metalwork *in situ* following first stage revision) in this setting leads to satisfactory union rates and infection eradication [13, 14]. In fact, it has been shown that union rates are comparable to those of aseptic revision cases [15]. Debate exists regarding whether ETO fixation should occur during the time of first or second stage revision. Positive results have been shown with delayed fixation (approximation of soft tissues without definitive fixation during the first stage revision) with regard to union rates [14]. Some have described fixation metalwork exchange at the time of second stage revision with good results. Fixation at the time of first-stage revision has shown not to have higher reinfection rates compared to patients without an ETO. [Shi] No clear consensus exists regarding the optimal timing of ETO fixation in a two-stage revision, but all appear to provide adequate results from the available literature.

3.4 Periprosthetic hip fracture

In the setting of periprosthetic hip fracture, ETO can be useful in the removal of well-fixed implants where revision is required. This is particularly useful in

Vancouver B2 and B3 fractures, where revision is generally indicated in a suitable patient. ETO allows for the removal of implants but also allows for the insertion of implants into the femoral diaphysis with improved visualisation. ETO can be performed through traditional techniques, although modifications have also been described that including ETO extension into the fracture fragment where appropriate [16]. Similar to other revision settings, ETO allows for more efficient removal of cement from the intramedullary canal. In the revision setting for fracture, a diaphyseal bearing stem is typically inserted where stem revision is required for a loose stem. ETO (along with the fracture itself) allows for direct visualisation of the distal canal into which the stem will be inserted. This allows for accurate sizing and reaming, allowing for optimal fit of the implanted stem. This may improve stem stability and help to reduce the rate of subsidence. Following this, the fracture fragments and ETO can be built around the stem and fixation is applied by the most suitable means.

3.5 Primary hip arthroplasty

While ETO is primarily considered in the revision setting, there have been reported cases of its utilisation of complex primary hip arthroplasty. Where conventional exposure techniques fail or when conventional stem placement techniques are not possible, ETO may play a role in the primary hip arthroplasty setting. Della Valle et al. initially described the use of ETO in complex primary surgery [17]. Indications for its use in their cohort were removal of hardware, complex femoral deformities and high-riding developmental hip dysplasia. They showed osteotomy healing rates of 80% (four of five cases) and highlighted the potential utility of ETO in selected complex primary cases. Wieser et al. later described the use of osteotomy in further complex primary settings including developmental dysplasia, high riding trochanter post perthes, post septic arthritis hip ankylosis, post-traumatic disturbed anatomy, avascular necrosis and osteoarthritis with severe varus abnormality [18]. While routine exposure techniques are suffice in majority of cases, the use of ETO can be of use in certain settings and should be considered in select cases.

4. Fixation techniques

Multiple ETO fragment fixation methods have been described including cables, wires, trochanteric plates and more novel techniques. Successful fixation ensures a high union rate and a low rate of proximal migration of the fragment in particular.

Cable fixation alone is a popular method of fixation. Cadaveric and biomechanical studies have shown promising results with regard to stability, which support its use. Generally, the osteotomy fragment is fixed with either two or three cables. Schwab et al. compared three cable versus two cable fixations and found no difference with regard to displacement, stiffness and peak force [19]. Previously, Chassin et al. (1997) proved that cable fixation with three cables following ETO in the setting of concomitant allograft bone packing and implant cementation showed no significant differences in stability compared to a non-osteotomised control femur [20]. More recently, Wyles et al. (2023) describe fixation with one or two cables distally to the lesser trochanter, one Luque wire above the lesser trochanter and one prophylactic cable distal to the osteotomy fragment. They recommend avoiding plate fixation unless absolutely necessary due to low rates of clinically significant fragment migration and concerns regarding symptomatic claw plates [21]. Overall, most would agree that cable fixation of the osteotomy fragment provides appropriate fixation in the majority of cases.

While previously popular, the use of wires alone has become less common due to concerns such as higher non-union rates and implant subsidence. Simank et al. showed an osteotomy non-union rate of 20% in their series and expressed concerns that this may potentially be secondary to the use of wires that were too thin [22]. Cables have become more favourable compared to wires in the majority of incidences. Prudhon et al. compared outcomes of fixation with cables, wires and plates and although there was a trend towards higher healing rates in plate fixation (88% in plate fixation, 82% with metallic wires, 70% with cables) although these findings were no statistically significant [23].

Zhu et al. (2013) biomechanically tested various ETO fragment fixation methods on cadaveric specimens including fixation with two wires, fixation with three wires, a short claw plate fixation with two wires and two cables, a short claw plate fixation with four cables and fixation with a long claw plate with four cables. They measured fragment translation with both vertical and lateral tension forces. They found that claw plate fixation methods had statistically significantly improved stability under these forces compared to wires alone [24].

There is debate around the use of trochanteric cable plate fixation following ETO. Supporters suggest that the plate system provides a stable construct with lower rates of proximal migration and high union rates. Sheridan et al. showed improved results using Dall-Miles plate fixation compared to cables alone in the setting of ETO for periprosthetic fracture revision. They showed improved clinical outcomes, radiological outcomes and lower rates of proximal fragment migration [25]. This was further supported, and some evidence suggests that trochanteric pain and limp were less following the use of a cable plate system. In cases of cables alone, there can be a slightly higher rate of proximal ETO migration. It is suggested that proximal migration can lead to abductor dysfunction and subsequent pain and limp. Proximal migration rates may be lower after using a cable plate fixation system. Concerns for trochanteric plates largely relate to symptoms including trochanteric pain and trochanteric bursitis, but there is evidence that this may not be the case, particularly with more modern plate systems [26]. Others also recommended the use of cable plate fixation in all cases, given advancements in plates and benefits as described [27].

Some more novel techniques have been described including the use of suture cord as described by Kuruvalli et al. (2008). This fixation technique describes the use of four strands of two vicryl formed into a single cord. Two drill holes are made in the osteotomy fragment through which the cord is passed and tied. They showed promising results including 19 of 20 patients having a bony union and proximal migration in only one patient [11]. This technique does not require the use of metalwork.

In complicated cases where there is significant proximal femur bone loss or fracture comminution, for example, bone graft in the form of cortical strut graft allograft may be utilised to provide further support to the cortex. Evidence has shown an increased cortex thickening following the integration of the strut graft, restoring bone loss [28]. Cortical strut grafts should generally only be used in cases of significant bone loss, however. There has been some evidence to suggest that healing rates can in fact be lower in cases where allograft has been used as part of the ETO fixation process, although this is debated.

There is debate as to the timing of ETO fixation and implant insertion. There are two known methods. First is the reconstitution method, whereby the ETO is fixed prior to implant insertion. This allows for easier anatomical fixation of the ETO fragment. Following this, the canal can be prepared. The second method is the scaffolding method, whereby the distal femur is prepared with the ETO open, and the ETO is fixed over the femoral implant after insertion. This allows for direct visualisation of the distal canal and accurate measuring/reaming, but on occasion, the ETO fragment may not anatomically reduce over the implant. Of course, if a cemented implant will be used, the reconstitution method will be required. Recent evidence has shown that in cadaveric studies, both techniques provide equal axial load stability [29]. Further studies should compare these techniques clinically.

Overall, there are multiple fixation methods. Most popular are the use of cables alone or cable plate constructs. Both have evidence to support their use. Decisions should be made on an individual basis. For example, cable plate constructs may be deemed appropriate in the setting of poor bone quality, comminution, osteotomy fragment fracture, revision for periprosthetic fracture or where cables alone may not provide adequate fixation. In other more routine cases, cables alone may be considered perfectly appropriate.

5. Prophylactic cables

The use of prophylactic cables is generally recommended. Cables are placed distal to the ETO site to prevent crack or fracture propagation to the femoral diaphysis, particularly when removing the stem and preparing the femur. Generally, the cable is placed after performing the osteotomy and prior to implant removal and femur preparation. In theory, it could be placed prior to the osteotomy if the precise distance of distal extension of ETO is known. Typically, the cable is placed approximately 1 cm distal to osteotomy.

6. Post-operative rehabilitation protocols

There is no clear consensus on post-operative protocols, and they differ between surgeons and institutions. Modern regimens largely suggest protected weight bearing with crutches/frames for varying periods. These periods differ and can be decided based on set time periods, symptoms or evidence of radiographic healing. Biomechanical studies have shown that the torsional strength of the osteotomised femur with an implant is 23% weaker than that of an implanted intact femur (cable fixation), and as such, protected weight bearing aims to reduce torsional stress and the associated risk of fracture. Many protocols advocate the avoidance of active abduction, which results in gluteal contraction, which may increase the risk of fragment proximal migration secondary to a vertical pull. The most consistent regimen consists of immediate mobilisation with protected weight bearing for 6–12 weeks (or full weight bearing for a further 6 weeks after an initial 6 weeks of protected weight bearing), avoiding active abduction exercises until 12 weeks post-operatively or until evidence of radiographic healing [4, 30].

7. Complications

There are well-described specific complications related to ETO. It is important to note, however, that the risk of iatrogenic femoral fracture (a complication of revision surgery without ETO) has shown to have poorer outcomes than patients who have undergone ETO. As such, this must be considered in revision cases [31]. A risk versus reward analysis of performing or not performing an ETO needs to be considered.

Of notable concern is the risk of non-union. In aseptic revision cases, union rates have been reported up to 100%. A recent systematic review showed union rates of 93.7% in aseptic revision cases [27]. Despite significant concerns for healing of the ETO fragment in the setting of infection, a recent systematic review showed ETO union rates of 95.1% and these concerns have largely been dispelled [32]. Of note, various techniques and fixation methods were used in the included studies. These results are reassuring, however, that successful outcomes in terms of union rates are likely even in the setting of revision for infection. Management of non-union is on a case-by-case basis, and there is limited literature that describes a treatment algorithm of approach. In the setting of a non-union with a loose femoral component, revision fixation +/− femoral component revision may be required. Asymptomatic non-union with a well-fixed stem may not require any further intervention.

Fracture of the ETO fragment intraoperatively is a well-known complication and was shown to occur in 4% of cases in a large study by Abdel et al. [33]. Fractures can occur at various points during the operation, including while performing the ETO, while removing cement or the stem, during trialling, during reduction or during broaching. Fractures of the ETO fragment can also occur post-operatively. In both cases, fractures of the shaft or greater trochanter can occur. Abdel et al. [33] showed a rate of 7% greater trochanter fracture in the post-operative period with a radiographic union rate of just 20%. Post-operative GT fracture does not appear to cause a significantly increased risk of dislocation. In cases of intra-operative ETO fragment fracture, the fracture should be initially reduced. In this setting, fixation with a cable plate construct may be considered if adequate fixation cannot be achieved with other methods to provide a more stable fixation construct. That said, there is no evidence to suggest that intra-operative ETO segment fracture affects the medium-term survival of the femoral implant (fluted tapered stems) [34]. In the case of post-operative ETO fragment fracture, each case requires individual assessment. If there is evidence of implant loosening, then further intervention may be required.

Subsidence of the femoral stem is seen in all revision settings including following ETO. Femoral stem subsidence can lead to complications such as the potential for increased dislocation rates, limb length changes and changes to abductor muscle tensioning. While there have been reported rates of stem subsidence of 16.6%, the majority of these are of less than 5 mm [34–36]. A recent systematic review showed a subsidence rate of >5 mm in 7.1% of cases [27]. Where a diaphyseal fixed stem is used following ETO, an opportunity is provided to directly visualise the femoral canal. This allows for accurate measurement and sizing of the femoral canal while allowing for direct visualisation while reaming. While this is important, stability is also closely related to the stem-cortex contact length, that is, the length of the stem within the femoral diaphysis. The greater the stem-cortex contact length, the greater the stability with axial loading [29]. In order to minimise subsidence, we should aim for a properly fitted stem with a long stem-to-cortex ratio.

Proximal migration of the ETO fragment can occur following ETO. It is more likely to occur in the setting of delayed union or non-union. The consequences of proximal migration can be non-union or disruption to abductor muscle function, leading to pain or an abnormal gait. An ETO, in comparison to other methods of trochanteric osteotomy, has inherent defensive mechanisms for migration. With a proper technique, the vastus lateralis and anterolateral muscles remain attached, which provide a contractile force to prevent migration. These attachments can also provide a compressive force across the ETO site to promote healing. There are a number of ways that we can try to reduce the risk of proximal migration. Firstly, it has been postulated that a longer osteotomy fragment leads to more muscle attachment and, therefore, more resistance to migration. In the post-operative period, limitation or inhibition of active or resisted hip abduction through appropriate instruction or bracing will lead to reduced abductor muscle firing. This should lead to less proximal pull on the ETO fragment. Some evidence suggests that the use of cable plate constructs or "claw plates" for ETO fixation can lead to reduced proximal migration rates in the setting of periprosthetic fracture [25]. Some have suggested more novel techniques such as the placement of a unicortical periprosthetic screw distal to one of the cerclage wires [37]. Overall through, proximal migration does not require further intervention in most cases, particularly where the distance is minimal [35].

Less specific to ETO but important potential complications include the risk of arterial or nerve injury if passing cables, dislocation, implant loosening and infection. All complications appear to have a higher rate in ETO used in periprosthetic fracture cases compared to aseptic revision cases. A systematic review has shown a dislocation rate of 3.7% (3.2% in periprosthetic fracture cases) and aseptic loosening of 1% (2.4% for periprosthetic fracture).

More recent evidence looking at ETO in the setting of revision for infection has shown promising results. While the complication rates following surgery for infected cases are generally higher than aseptic revision cases in general, there does not appear to be any increased risk of complications after the use of ETO specifically. This provides further support that its use in the setting of infection is safe where required [32].

8. Outcomes

Recent data shows that patients show improved post-operative outcomes following revision total hip replacement with ETO. PROMS are improved significantly post-operatively in the majority of cases, with evidence supporting similar outcomes to revisions that have not undergone ETO [38]. While there are multiple factors to patient satisfaction, results would suggest that ETO certainly does not seem to result in worse patient outcomes [38]. Outcomes following ETO can be considered closely linked to the indication for ETO in the first instance. Patients with periprosthetic fractures and infection are likely to have worse outcomes in settings with or without ETO, for example. Studies have compared the outcomes in patients who have had an unwanted intra-operative fracture compared to those who had an ETO performed and showed that outcomes were significantly better in the ETO group [31]. Overall, the outcomes following ETO are excellent, and there is no real evidence to suggest that the use of ETO in revision hip arthroplasty or certain periprosthetic fracture cases should be avoided.

Overall, ETO is an excellent option in multiple settings, particularly in revision hip arthroplasty. With proper technique, ETO facilitates implant removal, cement removal, acetabular exposure and femur reconstruction. The indications for its use continue to grow with time. The most recent evidence shows high union rates with low rates of complications, even in the settings of infection and cemented stems. As the technique continues to be refined and further evidence is revealed, outcomes will continue to improve. Importantly, its use should be individualised to each patient, and biomechanical principles should be adhered to at all times.

Author details

James Toale*, Mohamed Ahmed and James M. Broderick
Department of Trauma and Orthopaedics, St. Vincent's University Hospital, Dublin, Ireland

*Address all correspondence to: jamestoale@rcsi.ie

References

[1] Wagner H. A revision prosthesis for the hip joint. Der Orthopade. 1989;**18**(5):438-453

[2] Younger TI, Bradford MS, Magnus RE, Paprosky WG. Extended proximal femoral osteotomy: A new technique for femoral revision arthroplasty. The Journal of Arthroplasty. 1995;**10**(3):329-338

[3] Paprosky WG, Sporer SM. Controlled femoral fracture: Easy in. The Journal of Arthroplasty. 2003;**18**(3):91-93

[4] Chen WM, McAuley JP, Engh CA Jr, Hopper RH Jr, Engh CA. Extended slide trochanteric osteotomy for revision total hip arthroplasty. The Journal of Bone and Joint Surgery. 2000;**82**(9):1215

[5] Lakstein D, Kosashvili Y, Backstein D, Safir O, Lee P, Gross AE. The long modified extended sliding trochanteric osteotomy. International Orthopaedics. 2011;**35**:13-17

[6] Morcos MW, Decker MM, Lanting BA. Direct anterior approach for femoral component revision: Surgical technique for extended trochanteric osteotomy and anterior cortical window. Journal of Orthopaedics. 2020;**22**:274-277

[7] Bergemann R, Roytman GR, Ani L, Ramji AF, Leslie MP, Tommasini SM, et al. The feasibility of a novel 3D-printed patient specific cutting guide for extended trochanteric osteotomies. 3D Printing in Medicine. 2024;**10**(1):7

[8] Peters PC Jr, Head WC, Emerson RH Jr. An extended trochanteric osteotomy for revision total hip replacement. Journal of Bone and Joint Surgery. British Volume (London). 1993;**75**:158-159

[9] Charity J, Tsiridis E, Gusmão D, Bauze A, Timperley J, Gie G. Extended trochanteric osteotomy followed by cemented impaction allografting in revision hip arthroplasty. The Journal of Arthroplasty. 2013;**28**:154-160

[10] Huffman GR, Ries MD. Combined vertical and horizontal cable fixation of an extended trochanteric osteotomy site. The Journal of Bone and Joint Surgery. 2003;**85**(2):273-277

[11] Kuruvalli RR, Landsmeer R, Debnath UK, Suresh SP, Thomas TL. A new technique to reattach an extended trochanteric osteotomy in revision THA using suture cord. Clinical Orthopaedics and Related Research®. 2008;**466**(6):1444-1448

[12] Firestone TP, Hedley AK. Extended proximal femoral osteotomy for severe acetabular protrusion following total hip arthroplasty: A technical note. The Journal of Arthroplasty. 1997;**12**:344-345

[13] Levine BR, Della Valle CJ, Hamming M, Sporer SM, Berger RA, Paprosky WG. Use of the extended trochanteric osteotomy in treating prosthetic hip infection. The Journal of Arthroplasty. 2009;**24**(1):49-55

[14] Morshed S, Huffman GR, Ries MD. Extended trochanteric osteotomy for 2-stage revision of infected total hip arthroplasty. The Journal of Arthroplasty. 2005;**20**(3):294-301

[15] Cacciola G, Giustra F, Bosco F, Aprato A, De Meo F, Cavaliere P, et al. Extended trochanteric osteotomy is a safe procedure in two-stage hip revision: A systematic review of the literature. European Journal of

Orthopaedic Surgery & Traumatology. 2023;**33**(7):2695-2702

[16] Ladurner A, Zurmühle P, Zdravkovic V, Grob K. Modified extended trochanteric osteotomy for the treatment of Vancouver B2/B3 periprosthetic fractures of the femur. The Journal of Arthroplasty. 2017;**32**(8):2487-2495

[17] Della Valle CJ, Berger RA, Rosenberg AG, Jacobs JJ, Sheinkop MB, Paprosky WG. Extended trochanteric osteotomy in complex primary total hip arthroplasty: A brief note. The Journal of Bone and Joint Surgery. 2003;**85**(12):2385-2390

[18] Wieser K, Zingg P, Dora C. Trochanteric osteotomy in primary and revision total hip arthroplasty: Risk factors for non-union. Archives of Orthopaedic and Trauma Surgery. 2012;**132**:711-717

[19] Schwab JH, Camacho J, Kaufman K, Chen Q, Berry DJ, Trousdale RT. Optimal fixation for the extended trochanteric osteotomy: A pilot study comparing 3 cables vs 2 cables. The Journal of Arthroplasty. 2008;**23**(4):534-538

[20] Chassin EP, Silverton CD, Berzins A, Rosenberg AG. Implant stability in revision total hip arthroplasty: Allograft bone packing following extended proximal femoral osteotomy. The Journal of Arthroplasty. 1997;**12**(8):863-868

[21] Wyles CC, Hannon CP, Viste A, Perry KI, Trousdale RT, Berry DJ, et al. Extended trochanteric osteotomy in revision total hip arthroplasty. JBJS Essential Surgical Techniques. 2023;**13**(3):e21

[22] Simank HG, Chatzipanagiotis C, Kaps HP. Complication rate following trochanteric osteotomy in total hip endoprosthesis. A retrospective study with failure analysis. Zeitschrift fur Orthopadie und ihre Grenzgebiete. 1996;**134**(5):457-464

[23] Prudhon JL, Tardy N. Extended trochanteric osteotomy: Comparison of 3 modes of fixation: Metallic wires, cables, plate, about a series of 157 cases. SICOT-J. 2018;**4**:21

[24] Zhu Z, Ding H, Shao H, Zhou Y, Wang G. An in-vitro biomechanical study of different fixation techniques for the extended trochanteric osteotomy in revision THA. Journal of Orthopaedic Surgery and Research. 2013;**8**:1-7

[25] Sheridan GA, Galbraith A, Kearns SR, Curtin W, Murphy CG. Extended trochanteric osteotomy (ETO) fixation for femoral stem revision in periprosthetic fractures: Dall–miles plate versus cables. European Journal of Orthopaedic Surgery & Traumatology. 2018;**28**:471-476

[26] Zhang B, Du Y, Zhang Y, Dong Y, Zhang T, Zhou Y. Comparison of functional and radiographic outcomes between two fixation methods for extended trochanteric osteotomy in revision total hip arthroplasty: A retrospective cohort study. The Journal of Arthroplasty. 2022;**37**(9):1844-1850

[27] Malahias MA, Gkiatas I, Selemon NA, De Filippis R, Gu A, Greenberg A, et al. Outcomes and risk factors of extended trochanteric osteotomy in aseptic revision total hip arthroplasty: A systematic review. The Journal of Arthroplasty. 1 Nov 2020;**35**(11):3410-3416

[28] Lim CT, Amanatullah DF, Huddleston JI III, Hwang KL, Maloney WJ, Goodman SB. Use of cortical strut allograft after extended trochanteric osteotomy in revision total hip arthroplasty. The Journal of Arthroplasty. 2017;**32**(5):1599-1605

[29] Tarity TD, Xiang W, Gkiatas I, Meyers KN, Malahias MA, Rodriguez JA, et al. Extended trochanteric osteotomy closure performed before or after canal preparation and stem impaction does not affect axial stability. The Journal of Arthroplasty. 2022;**37**(8):S964-S970

[30] Sambandam SN, Duraisamy G, Chandrasekharan J, Mounasamy V. Extended trochanteric osteotomy: Current concepts review. European Journal of Orthopaedic Surgery & Traumatology. 2016;**26**:231-245

[31] Lerch M, Von Lewinski G, Windhagen H, Thorey F. Revision of total hip arthroplasty: Clinical outcome of extended trochanteric osteotomy and intraoperative femoral fracture. Technology and Health Care. 2008;**16**(4):293-300

[32] Almaslmani S, Entezari B, Safir OA, Gross AE, Kuzyk PR. Clinical and functional outcomes of extended trochanteric osteotomy in 2-stage revision Total hip arthroplasty for periprosthetic joint infection: A systematic review and meta-analysis. The Journal of Arthroplasty. 2023;**38**(9):1900-1907

[33] Abdel MP, Wyles CC, Viste A, Perry KI, Trousdale RT, Berry DJ. Extended trochanteric osteotomy in revision total hip arthroplasty: Contemporary outcomes of 612 hips. The Journal of Bone and Joint Surgery. 2021;**103**(2):162-173

[34] Garabano G, Gessara AM, Pesciallo CA, Alamino LP, Del Sel H. Extended trochanteric osteotomy (ETO) and fluted tapered modular stems in revision hip arthroplasty. Does ETO integrity for consolidation, really matter? Journal of Orthopaedics. 2021;**23**:250-255

[35] Hamad K, Konan S. Extended trochanteric osteotomy in revision hip arthroplasty: A case series study and systematic literature review. Art. 2022;**4**(1):14

[36] Kang PD, Pei FX, Shen B, Zhou ZK, Yang J. Extended trochanteric osteotomy for removal of solidly-fixed femoral implants in total hip revision. Zhonghua Wai Ke Za Zhi. 2009;**47**(3):177-180

[37] Ismailidis P, Mündermann A, Stoffel K. A Monocortical screw for preventing trochanteric escape in extended trochanteric osteotomy: A simple solution to a complicated problem? Journal of Clinical Medicine. 2023;**12**(8):2947

[38] Jopek T, Chodór P, Łapaj Ł, Woźniak W, Michalak S, Kruczyński J. Extended trochanteric osteotomy does not compromise functional and radiographic outcomes of femoral stem revisions with the use of an Uncemented modular conical stem. Journal of Clinical Medicine. 2024;**13**(19):5921

Chapter 6

Rehabilitation of the Hip

Rodrigo Hamada and Gustavo Enrique Barros

Abstract

Although we are currently seeing increasing progress in the scientific literature on the intervention of physiotherapy and rehabilitation in the management of groin-related pathologies, through the formation of working groups with specialists in the field and the development of clinical guidelines and consensus on the management specifically of femoroacetabular friction syndrome (FAI), there is still a paucity of information on how to treat individuals with micro-hip instability in a non-invasive manner. While orthopedic surgeons are currently focusing on solving these problems with increasingly sophisticated and less invasive surgical techniques, rehabilitators believe that conservative treatment may benefit these patients and thus avoid and/or delay hip arthroplasty. This chapter will describe a preventive neuromuscular re-education approach based on proprioceptive control with promising results in this type of patient, as well as, in a second part, the rehabilitative management once the patient has undergone primary hip arthroplasty, based on the existing scientific literature, which is very extensive, with internationally validated successful results.

Keywords: microinestability of the hip, FAI, proprioceptive reeducation, total hip arthroplasty (THR), rehabilitation

1. Introduction

The growing scientific evidence on groin pain has led scientists to develop different treatment algorithms based on international classifications of the pathology. In addition, magnetic resonance imaging as a method of soft tissue imaging and the increasing development of arthroscopic techniques with new surgical approach portals have meant that entities such as femoroacetabular friction syndrome (FAI) and labral lesions are now considered as sources of groin pain and are included within specific hip injuries when using the Doha classification of groin pain [1]. Femoroacetabular impingement is understood as an undesired contact with the anatomy that occurs because of the impact observed between the femoral components, specifically areas of the femoral neck, and the external lip of the acetabular labrum, generating micro-injuries at the soft parts of this joint. Femoroacetabular impingement can be differentiated in lesions where there is an abnormal morphology of the neck and/or femoral head, CAM type lesions, in those lesions where an excessive acetabular coverage of the femoral head is observed, called PINCER type or a combination of both called mixed type.

It is believed that the bony deformity progresses toward degeneration of the acetabular labrum, generating changes in the pressures and loads on the articular cartilage, which would lead to osteoarthritic changes throughout life [2]. Philippon et al. and McCarthy et al. pointed to abnormal joint morphology as the most common cause of labral pathology [3]. Ryan, Julianne & als. conducted a systematic review to identify and examine the risk factors for groin/hip injuries in field sports (FBS). They conducted a literature search of 14 electronic databases using keywords. What these authors did was to include those studies that met the selected criteria considering the chosen risk factors for hip injuries in those field sports that exhibited injuries. Risk factors identified were previous injuries, older age, body mass index (BMI), weakness of the hip adductor muscles (WHAM), early biological maturation, smaller diameter of the dominant femur, decreased total range of motion (TROM) of the hip, and varying strength ratios of hip muscle groups (hip abduction and adduction with rotation and bilateral difference in maximal extension torque) [4]. Lewis et al. assume in this study that the muscles that should control the stability of the hip are often insufficient, and this would lead to micro-injuries in the soft tissues of the joint. For non-specialists, it can take up to 3.1 years to determine whether a hip pathology is present [5].

Although current diagnoses are based on clinical-radiological findings, there are no articles that show as evidence that groin pain associated with hip pathology is generated by alterations in the lack of control of the forces exerted on the hip. Several authors have reported good-to-excellent clinical results after arthroscopic decompression of the FAI and the labral fixation. Although literature reviews with low-level evidence support arthroscopic surgery for FAI correction and stabilization of labral tears, there is still no relevant randomized controlled trial research comparing and favoring the choice of surgical versus nonsurgical treatment in this population. There is a growing body of literature describing postoperative rehabilitation following arthroscopic hip procedures [5].

At the same time, the concept of hip micro-instability is growing in the scientific community, and even more so in the young, athletic population, an entity that is based on an altered proprioceptive component which would lead to joint degeneration over the years.

2. Functional anatomy

The hip joint is of the diarthrodial type with three degrees of freedom of movement, consisting of the proximal end of the femur and the cotyloid socket belonging to the ilium of the pelvis. When any nosological entity affects the functionality of the hip, fundamental activities such as dressing, hygiene, walking, or more demanding activities such as running, jumping, or even going up and down stairs are affected [6]. Bolia, Ioana et al. [7] define hip instability as "an extraphysiological movement that causes pain with or without symptoms of joint instability." They suggest that criteria for defining hip micro-instability have not yet been proposed [7]. They also argue that repetitive rotation and axial loading could trigger symptoms. Therefore, they claim that this biomechanical alteration could put the soft tissues of the hip joint at risk by generating groin pain [7].

Retchford and cols [8] theorize that in the human body there are two muscular systems: local and global. They suggest that local muscles are responsible for providing joint stability by acting close to the joint axis, predominantly providing joint compression rather than torsion, and could stiffen the joint due to their extensive insertions into the key passive elements of the joint. In contrast, global muscles are superficial muscles, which can generate greater joint torque due to their larger physiological cross-sectional area (PCSA) and greater moment arm. There are numerous studies on pathological muscle function and dysfunction in the lumbar spine, cervical spine, knee, and pelvis. These investigations have identified local muscle dysfunctions in people with pain and pathologies, and it was seen that specific muscle retraining can restore muscle function [8].

We have found very little evidence of muscle action in relation to dynamic control of the hip, and how its stabilizing action might slow the progression of a joint disruption. Cassartelli et al. [9] found that patients with symptomatic FAI had significant muscle weakness for all hip muscle groups except the internal rotators and extensors. Of those articles suggesting that muscle hypofunction may be implicated in the progression of joint pathology, most were conducted with patients who had some degree of joint degeneration, such as osteoarthritis of the hip (OA). Therefore, more scientific evidence is needed to substantiate that preventive muscle re-education works at an early age through physiotherapy protocols can successfully influence the control of forces that displace the proximal femur in relation to the acetabulum [8].

Some hip muscles support the hip joint capsule. More specifically, the iliocapsularis muscles, the deep fibers of the iliopsoas, the quadratus femoris, gemelli, obturator internus and externus, gluteus minimus, and the indirect reflex tendon of the rectus femoris are the main stabilizers of the femoral head.

The iliocapsularis muscle originates from the anteromedial hip capsule and the anteroinferior iliac spine (AIIS). In relation to its contribution to the support of the hip capsule, the iliocapsularis has the greatest contribution as it attaches at the 2:30 o'clock position [10]. In their study, Ward et al. argue that the insertion of the iliocapsularis muscle originates in the hip joint capsule and suggest that its contraction could tighten the anterior part of the capsule, which would help to stabilize the femoral head in dysplastic acetabulae [10]. With this theory, they suggest that repetitive use of this muscle would explain its hypertrophy in dysplastic hips and its atrophy in stable hips [10]. In the *article* by Neuman [11], it is stated that the tendon of the iliacus muscle, at distal level, and the psoas run anterior and medial to the femoral head, going to its distal insertion in the lesser trochanter. This tendon, wide, presents a posterior deviation of 35° to 45° more or less, and crosses the pubic ramus on its superior aspect. If the hip is fully extended, the lever of the muscle to flex the hip is increased because the angle of insertion of the tendon is raised, and if the hip is at 90, this lever is increased [11]. This parallel increase in the lever when the hip increases, the flexion angles compensates for the loss of muscle power in the active work of the muscle, which is marked by the decrease in its length. If the bilateral contraction is isolated, any muscle performing hip flexion should rotate the femur toward the ilium, as well as the pelvis over the femur, and perhaps both actions simultaneously. Neuman argues that the external rotator muscles pass postero-lateral to the axis of longitudinal (or vertical) rotation of the coxofemoral joint anatomical position. Since this axis of rotation, which is vertical, remains aligned to the femur, he suggests that only in the anatomical position is it truly vertical. It only considers as stabilizing muscles from the femur to the pelvis (and vice versa), the geminus (superior and inferior), obturator internus, and quadratus cruris. These three external rotators, together with the gluteus maximus, the pyramidalis of the pelvis are the primary ones. The secondary ones, from the anatomical position, are the posterior fibers of the gluteus medius, gluteus minimus, obturator externus, sartorius, and the long portion of the biceps femoris [11]. If the hip is placed with a few degrees of internal rotation, the line of force of the obturator externus muscle, passing through the longitudinal axis, will not be able to generate force in the horizontal plane. The external rotators, having a nearly horizontal line of force (except for the pelvic pyramid), produce effective hip external rotation because almost *all* the force generated is used to torque the joint and coapt the articular surfaces involved. In the same way as the external rotators of the shoulder (infraspinatus and *teres* minor), these external rotators of the hip provide the necessary stability for the articular centering of the coxofemoral [11].

Orthopedic surgeons at our *hospital* prefer the posterolateral approach for hip prosthesis placement. Tsai et al. demonstrated the importance of preserving the anatomy of the hip joint capsule. They were able to corroborate that suturing the joint capsule after hip replacement, even without suturing the external rotators, significantly reduced posterior dislocations of primary replacements [12]. It is therefore critical that orthopedic surgeons, in addition to repairing the capsular component, also suture the rotator muscles because of their important proprioceptive role and thus decrease the incidence of posterior dislocation.

Khan et al. recommend careful repair of posterior structures when using the posterior approach to reduce the risk of dislocation [13].

There are activities such as sudden changes of direction, braking, and sudden fixation of the lower limb on the ground where the importance of the contraction of the external rotators to perform the rotation of the trunk and pelvis is observed, taking a fixed point at the hip. For example, if the right lower limb is fixed on the ground, the muscular contraction of the external rotators can rotate the pelvis and trunk to the left, as well as a contraction of the gluteus maximus could extend and externally rotate the right hip, giving the necessary thrust to change the direction of movement and propel. This is a clear example of the muscular stability of the external rotators at the hip in activities involving high velocities [11].

Some authors describe the greater trochanter of the femur with four facets for the insertion of the gluteal mantle (anterior, lateral, posterior, and a superoposterior facet), and where the gluteus medius muscle would be in the lateral and superoposterior facets, leaving the anterior facet to the gluteus minimus [14]. In turn, of the existing hip pouches, the trochanteric pouch is responsible for covering the posterior facet as well as part of the lateral insertion of the gluteus medius muscle. The medial subgluteal bursa is located below the gluteus medius tendon and covers the superior portion of the lateral facet, and the minimal subgluteal bursa is located on the anterior facet below the gluteus minimus tendon, medial to its insertion, extending medially to cover the anterior part of the joint capsule [14].

As we know, in the depth of the gluteal mantle we have the lesser of them, which *is in* front of the medial one and that goes to the greater trochanter to insert in the antero-lateral face of the same [11]. Secondarily, by means of its distal tendon that reaches the anterosuperior capsule of the hip, when extreme articular movements are produced, they retract the capsule and avoid many times the pinching of the same one. Continuing with the anatomy of the gluteus minimus, Neuman maintains that it represents approximately 20% of the total group that abducts the hip in transverse section. Since it has three sets of fibers, all of them perform abduction, with the anterior fibers contributing to internal rotation (more if combined with flexion), while the posterior fibers perform secondary external rotation [11]. Finally, Kumagai et al. suggest that the gluteus minimum together with the gluteus medius plays a fundamental role in gait by stabilizing the pelvis [15].

Other authors through cadaveric studies were concerned with the rectus femoris of the thigh correlating different strain injuries in the findings of the anatomy of the muscle, and corroborated these injuries in sports activities such as sprints or throws in sports such as soccer. The rectus femoris muscle is usually described as a bipennate structure with two heads of origin (direct, or straight, from the anteroinferior iliac spine and indirect, or reflex, from the superior acetabular crest). These proximal tendons extend distally one third of the length of the muscle belly while remaining superficial to the ventral surface of the muscle. Similarly, the distal tendon extends along the distal two thirds of the muscle belly and lie superficial to the dorsal surface of the muscle. The muscle fibers arise from the proximal tendons and extend both medially and laterally in the distal direction to terminate at the distal tendon of insertion, thus giving rise to the bipennate structure of the muscle [16].

2.1 Physical examination

We begin the physical examination of the patient by evaluating his or her general appearance, since this may provide us with clues as to the origin of the pain. Then, we start the examination in standing position, since the hip is a component of the kinematic chain of the lower limb, we will receive the most information in the loading activities. For this purpose, we will evaluate the Trendelenburg test in static, the alignment, the articular laxity tests, and the gait in dynamic. Domb et al. [17] consider the Trendelenburg test positive when the pelvis sinks more than 2 cm, while the patient lifts the contralateral limb off the ground. When lifting the right leg, the abductor musculature that is under load is being tested; therefore, a positive sign suggests abductor insufficiency. The maneuver should be performed first on the unaffected side to establish a comparative standard [17].

If we find any discrepancy either true or false in the length of the legs, we have several ways to corroborate it, even more so when we see an alteration in gait due to a shorter limb [17]. We begin the examination by comparing by observing the height of the shoulder girdle in relation to the ipsilateral hemipelvis. From there, we check whether there is an inclination of the pelvis because if present it can generate a discrepancy in length and then, it is appropriate to measure the distance from the anterior superior iliac spine (ASIS) to the internal malleolus of the limb. If alterations are found in the measurement, we will define this situation as a real discrepancy at the length of the limb being an alteration in the bony proportion of the limbs. If we do not find a real discrepancy and we observe an alteration in the gait due to a shorter limb, it may be due to some other alterations such as scoliosis, pelvic alterations or retractions, and/or muscular contractures that affect the position of the pelvis in space [17]. Therefore, it is appropriate to evaluate the spine from the inspection in several positions. One would be in standing position, asking the patient to flex the trunk anteriorly, and the observer from behind observes the alignment of the spinous processes of the spine to rule out any anomaly at the three axes of space. Then, we evaluate the sagittal plane and pay attention to the curves presented by the patient, since contractures of the hip flexors can generate a lumbar hyperlordosis, while a marked paravertebral contracture will generate an abnormal tension that will affect the coxofemoral [17].

Whittle et al. [18] suggest that no one gait is the same as another, and although there are standard evaluation patterns and although muscle activity is one of the fundamental components of gait, to define a movement *pattern,* we know that the interaction of other anatomical elements such as bone, joint, and nervous system is necessary. There are variables that are used to define a normal gait [18]. Normal gait requires that each lower limb, when bearing weight, should not be overcome, and should be able to maintain a balance on a single limb both statically and dynamically. In turn, the lower limb that is balancing must be able to finish that phase and prepare to go for heel strike, with the general muscular component of the lower limb having the ability to be able to perform the various gait cycles [18]. Naturally, the gait cycles should be performed as naturally as possible, with a minimum energetic cost to be as economical as possible [18]. Abnormal gait patterns are often identified by simple observation and, in other cases by means of a validated instrument, detect functional and/or anatomical anomalies that often lead to the use of external supports to alleviate the high energetic cost [18]. Disorders of the central nervous system, peripheral nervous system, control centers, and other structures that govern the other components of movement (bones, muscles, joints, etc.) are a challenge for rehabilitators, since these types of conditions are often irreversible and leave great sequelae in patients [18].

In seated position, the evaluation is done bilaterally, first evaluating the circulatory system, checking the normal existence of the dorsal, pedial, and posterior tibial pulses, and then inspecting the condition of the skin and lymph nodes around the hip. The assessment of the ROM of hip rotations we prefer to do according to Domb et al. [17], where the sitting position with the pelvis fixed in the plane and the hip in 90 degrees of flexion avoids variations in the arc of flexion. The range of hip internal rotation is 20° to 35° and the external rotation is 30° to 70°. Loss of internal rotation is one of the early signs of problems such as arthritis, osteoarthrosis, joint effusion, slippage of the femoral epiphysis, and muscle contractures [17].

Special maneuvers are included in the supine assessment. There are a few special maneuvers to perform on the hip. We use three maneuvers recommended by Hoppe and col. [19] that we interpret as the most sensitive and specific for hip micro-instability. They are as follows:

- The first one is performed in lateral decubitus, with the patient's affected limb on top. We place the hip in abduction from 30 to 45 degrees approximately, while we extend and externally rotate it, and at the same time the greater trochanter is pushed from posterior to forward. If the patient refers pain in the anterior aspect of the hip, the test is positive [19]. This test is called AB-HEER.

- The second test is in prone position and evaluates hip instability, hence its name. The patient's limb is rotated outward, while the operator pushes into the plane of the greater trochanter on its posterior aspect. The presence of pain in the anterior aspect of the hip is taken as a positive result of the test [19].

- The third test is called the anterior apprehension test. This test is performed with the patient in the supine position, with the legs hanging and the operator at the foot of the examination table. An anterior force is applied to the hip to be evaluated (hyperextending the hip and externally rotating it at the same time), while the contralateral hip is held by the patient in maximum flexion. If the patient manifests any painful symptom, we consider it as positive. It is called HEER test [19].

2.2 Proprioception

For adequate functional joint stability to exist, the components must be able to adapt and be flexible to the demands as these demands vary from individual to individual. The articular stability is maintained by means of the constituent elements of the sector such as the static and dynamic components of the joint [20]. Within the passive ones, we can name those tissues with a large connective component such as ligaments, articular capsules, articular cartilage added to the conformation of the articular surfaces and the forces with which it must interact (e.g., friction) [20]. The dynamic oversees the muscular structure, which must have a back and forth with the nervous system, to achieve dynamic stability in the different activities. We include here the articular range, the components of the force (pure force, resistance, and power) and the proprioceptive system, meaning the recognition of the articular position [20].

Mechanoreceptor afferent appears to provide critical information to the central nervous system regarding joint movement and position, and results in muscle stabilization that is essential for functional activities [20]. It is relevant to understand the importance of proprioception in the stabilization of the joint, since it is not only anatomical problems that lead the patient to develop degenerative processes in the joint, but also the alteration of this permanent information system that allows us an adequate function [21]. All activities require situational awareness, with a wide field of attention to continuously monitor the environment, filter irrelevant information, and simultaneously execute complex motor programs [21].

In 1900, Erwin Payr hypothesized the existence of the protective ligament-muscular reflex, where ligaments, bones, muscles, and receptors act synergistically to provide safety and stable motion to a given joint. Saccomani et al. defined the proprioception as that variation of the sensory modality of touch, which is specialized and involves the sensation of movement and the recognition of joint position [22]. It is composed of three elements such as the awareness of static joint position, the conscious detection of movement and acceleration, and an efferent action of a circuit that initiates the reflex response and controls the muscular activity.

Therefore, we believe that stimulating the dynamic stability of the hip decreases the loads on the joint leading to an alleviation of symptoms and delaying any degenerative process. Some authors recommend not producing interruptions in therapeutic exercise therapies, since they consider that if these do not have the adequate duration (at least 12 weeks) or if after having completed a prudential time of training (3 months) and the expected recovery levels were not reached; the evolution could be related to poor or bad results [23]. In relation to this, there are data that suggest that after training for 6 weeks, the considered good results were 48%, and this percentage rose to 68% if the training stimuli reached 12 weeks, having as the most significant parameters pain and joint function, which only improved after that time (12 weeks) [23]. Therefore, training programs should exceed 6 weeks of stimulation *to* generate the neuromuscular changes necessary to achieve dynamic joint stability [23].

The proprioceptive re-education treatment plan that we carried out on our patients lasted 120 days, that is, 4 months. The treatment frequency used was three times a week, each session lasting 1 hour. The treatment was divided into the following stages:

1. Static stability stage for in-office exercise.

2. Dynamic stability stage for exercise in the gymnasium.

3. Stage of stability to the usual effort in the field.

4. Stability stage of effort stability for normal activity in the field.

Throughout the protocol, an approach based on proprioceptive reeducation is sought, without leaving aside the symptomatic treatment when the patient needs it. Physical agents are applied according to the pain and inflammation according to each stage, as well as the manual therapy approach indicated to achieve relaxation and analgesia.

For the conformation of the proprioceptive reeducation protocol, we seek that the characteristics of the exercises for the specific training of proprioception seek:

- Achieve dynamic stabilization of the joints, in the face of rapid and abrupt movements.
- Determine a correct muscular balance between agonists, antagonists, and synergist (elongation—strength).
- To automate specific gestures [24]

3. Proprioceptive treatment protocol

In this first stage of static stability, we focus on the recognition of the articular position, always respecting the patient's clinical condition (**Table 1**). As a first step, we focus on the initial examination and corroborate that the patient is not undergoing any acute process, because if so, the first objective would be to control pain and inflammation. For this, we use the physical agents available to modulate the inflammatory processes, and we indicate a relative rest but without neglecting the functional activities that can be performed without overloading the tissues under repair, and if necessary, we will rely on some external support.

Regarding the range of motion (ROM), the objective of this stage is to limit it to ranges where the joint is maintained in a position of capsular looseness, thus allowing an optimal joint filling volume and thus minimizing the nociceptive afferences produced by the microtraumas that are generated when the activities exceed the normal joint ranges. In case the joint is very symptomatic, we apply manual therapy to generate analgesia and capsular relaxation, combining passive and active-assisted techniques (mobilizations with movement). Then, we use stretching as a resource to flex the shortened dynamic stabilizers.

We start at this stage the restoration of the normal lumbopelvic movement since it is often altered due to pain and the predominance that we observe in the mobilizing muscles over the primary stabilizers. We then work on muscle balance by emphasizing the primary stabilizers of the anterior displacement of the femoral head on the acetabulum. We start the work of proprioceptive re-education following the child's neurodevelopment guidelines. Learning and mastering motor development activities is an indispensable factor for everyday physiological movements (head, control, sitting, rolling, quadruped, and standing with two legs). For this reason, works carried out in closed kinetic chain (CKC) optimize the activity of the muscle groups involved in this activity by generating muscular co-contraction, achieving stabilization and joint centering, which is the key to reducing the loads on a given point of the articular cartilage, thus reducing the possibility of degeneration. This then allows the use of the open kinetic chain (OKC) essential for movement. This means that the therapy itself

Phases of treatment	Objectives	Treatment
Static stability stage for office exercise. (from 0 to 3 weeks)	**Decrease pain and inflammation** **ROM CONTROL:** • Retrieve the hip extension. • Limit hip flexion between 90° and 100°. • ADD-ABD: 0°–30°. • Hip rotations of hip: o RE: 0°–30°. o RI: 0°–15°. • **Maintain adequate tone of the muscles stabilizing primary** • **Starts with proprioceptive activities** • **Gait reeducation** • **Patient education in ADLS**	• Regulated cryotherapy [25] • Relative rest • Walking aid (crutches) to reduce symptoms of ambulation • Manual Therapy: Distal and lateral traction to treat Kaltenborn grades I and II pain [26]. • Mobilization with motion (MWM): MWM lateral distraction in supine, distal traction in prone for rectus femoris (RF) [27]. • Selective stretching of psoas, iliocapsularis, Tensor de la fascia Lata (TFL), hamstrings, rectus femoris, abdominal muscles [28]. • Restore correct lumbopelvic rhythm [29]. • Selective muscle strengthening of the psoasiliac, abductors, adductors, external rotators, gluteus maximus, CORE muscles, spinal, iliocapsularis, rectus femoris, TFL, and hamstrings. CORE work [30]. • Proprioceptive work: Normalize muscular and articular restrictions: muscular inhibition + articular re-centering. Recognition of joint position. • Limit repetitive microtrauma caused by movements up to or beyond the joint limits generating repetitive injuries or plastic elongation of the joint capsule (this would increase the forces on the other static stabilizers). • Rhythmic stabilization techniques seeking static isometry at different degrees of joint movement. • Gait pattern reeducation: Reduce the gait stride length of the affected hip with emphasis on dynamic stretching of the anterior flexors. • Decrease or abolish prolonged deep flexion postures (do not sit on soft surfaces (soft armchairs, hammocks, etc.), do not cross your legs or pivot on that hip). • Limit straight leg elevation (SLR).

Table 1.
Proprioceptive re-education protocol—Stage I: Static stability stage for office-based exercise.

should start in a relatively easy position for the activation of the muscle chains by applying stimuli to the mechanoreceptors, the starting position being supine.

Gait re-education is a key factor in the rehabilitation of these patients as it involves working both open and closed movement chains. Gait training exercises, such as step training over obstacles of different heights (cone exercises), are started prenatally to develop symmetry between the lower extremities. Symmetrical flexion of the hip, knee, and ankle over the obstacle produces motor control of the muscles of the entire limb receiving the load, and symmetry of the triceps suralis (gastrocnemius/soleus) during the push-off and equal support time between the limbs are vital components of this work. We then break down the different phases of gait and re-educate those muscles that are functioning inadequately, considering the three planes of space, with progressive progressions of difficulty. Finally, at this stage we instruct the patient to abolish those postures and/or activities that predispose the hip joint to abnormal movement patterns (**Table 2**).

In this second stage of the dynamic stability protocol to exercise in the gym, regarding pain and inflammation management, we continued with physical agents and analytical manual therapy to reduce as much as possible the nociception generated in the re-education work. Dry needling techniques together with electroanalgesia have given us the best results, as well as manual therapy with oscillations in degrees I and II to mitigate pain and allow capsuloligamentary relaxation. Since at this stage of re-education the patient should already have fully recovered joint range of motion (ROM), we do not focus on the patient demonstrating an adequate mechanical gait

Phases of treatment	Objectives	Treatment
Stage of dynamic stability to exercise in the gym. (3 to 6 weeks).	• **Pain and inflammation management as needed** • **Full ROM in active and passive** • **Start of activities proprioceptive activities dynamics** • **Avoid offsets and possible tendinopathies of synergists** • **Increase general muscular endurance**	• Selective electroanalgesia + dry needling on muscle trigger points [31]. • Manual therapy: distal and lateral traction to treat pain. • Mobilization with movement (MWM): Lateral distraction MWM in supine for internal rotation and for external rotation. • Selective flexibility of muscle chains (emphasis on flexor group). • Concentric/excentric analytical strengthening of iliocapsularis, gluteus maximus and gluteus medius, and internal/external rotators. Inhibit overactivation of hip flexors. • Dynamic proprioceptive work: • Seeking mental representation and awareness of the position of the pelvis in relation to the femur the position of the pelvis in relation to the femur by means of the muscle contractions in open and closed chains of closed chains of movements. • Distinguish hip flexion from lumbar flexion. • Start with basic squat exercises: bring the buttocks backwards and not forwards (not forward). Buttocks backwards and not forward (sit on a low stool). • Gluteal activation (abd + rot ext). • Once control of the squat has been achieved, move on to the single leg squat, aiming to abolish knee valgus. • Awareness of Hurdle step control (step over obstacle). • Achieve rotational control of the body in quadruped. • Re-educate normal and athletic gait on treadmill without incline.

Table 2.
Proprioceptive re-education protocol—Stage II: Dynamic stability stage to exercise in the gym.

pattern without compensations. Here, we have had good results with the incorporation of race walking as an activity to coordinate postural gestures with speed.

Here, we start the bipodal exercises in load such as the use of the squat. First, we allow the patient to do it in the position that is most favorable to him/her and to then generate load to the hip flexor component (gluteus and hamstrings) and then, we take the trunk more toward extension to overload both quadriceps. Once the patient achieves this, we move on to the lunges work, first looking for the patient to master the sagittal plane (anteroposterior imbalances) and then incorporating the frontal plane (toward the sides), leaving the axial plane for the end, since it is the most complex of all. Each of these tasks is initiated first on a solid surface to seek control on unstable surfaces in a second instance (**Table 3**).

At this stage, all activities are carried out at the extremes of the joint range, to progressively stimulate the control of the stabilizers of the anterior displacement of the femoral head in its eccentric component. Here, we introduce exercises where patients should progress more toward the associative phase of motor learning, with greater task complexity and a focus on generating neuromuscular solutions that minimize error without focusing solely on movement. This may include a greater emphasis on visual distraction and/or working memory, as well as perturbation training during dynamic exercise such as seeking stability on unstable platforms with distractors such as catching and/or throwing a ball, controlling the upper body in the face of unbalancing forces and other situations where stability is disturbed.

We also incorporate bipodal and unipodal plyometric tasks combined with different heights and types of jumps. Here, we also intensify muscular balance through work involving concentric-eccentric activity of the stabilizers to achieve automatic and involuntary joint centering in dynamic activities. We focus the work on the control of the pelvis in relation to the femur in closed chains of movement so that later, in open chains of movement, the patient can differentiate the movement of the femur on the pelvis and vice versa (**Table 4**).

At this last stage, patients are encouraged to perform activities that develop skills resembling their normal activities. They are programmed with a series of activities for

Stage of stability to the usual effort in the field (6 to 9 weeks).	• **Full ROM active and passive in dynamic activities.** • **Increase activities at all levels planes of movement.** • **Agility drills with hip pivots hip pivots.**	• Full ROM of the limb (pivoting at the end ranges of the joint arc). • Moderate proprioceptive exercises and activities under load. • Incorporate unstable planes (medicine ball). • Achieve correct total deep squat. • Progress from light jogging to medium, ¾ and maximum speed. • Bipodal and monopodal jumping and landing [32]. • Specific proprioceptive exercises in load at the extremes of the ROM. • Descending stairs in light race walking, jogging, and medium speed. • Jumping in all directions bipodal and monopodal.

Table 3.
Proprioceptive reeducation protocol—Stage II: Stage of stability to the usual effort in the field.

Stress stability stage for normal field activity. (9 to 12 weeks).	**Priorities performance agility and correct sporting gestures** • **Testing of progression of activities in speed medium, ¾ and maximum speed.**	• Incorporate speed activities as they involve a good contraction/relaxation relationship in muscle function as agonist/antagonist, synergist, and concurrent synergist. • Incorporation of sport specific elements as part of movement re-education. • Agility drills in the field: lateral movements at medium and maximum speed, without and with obstacles [33]. • Moderate to high intensity plyometrics. • Jumping in all directions. • Incorporate contact activities with opponents.

Table 4.
Proprioceptive re-education protocol—Stage 4: Effort stability stage for normal field activity.

increasing complexity with different types of disturbing elements. We have also had good results using unstable platforms with multimedia technology through virtual reality, where we try to get the patient to focus their vision and hearing on a device, while the therapist generates external stimuli on the platform so that they develop unconscious control mechanisms, imitating the activities they will be subjected to when they are discharged from kinesics. Finally, the combination of different types of jumping, with bipodal and monopodal landing from the plane and then from different heights, seeks body control and minimizing reaction time when falling.

3.1 Outcome measures

In our Kinesiology Unit, we opted for the Copenhagen Hip and Groin Outcome Score (HAGOS), which was proposed as a score to measure the results that the patient answers by means of a questionnaire, following standards based on the consensus for the selection of Health Measurement Instruments (COSMIN) [34]. This questionnaire is fundamentally designed for those young middle-aged individuals who are active, that is, in acceptable physical condition, but who for some reason present groin or hip symptoms of variable duration. This scale evaluates separately the pain, those symptoms referred to the groin area, what physical function they present in daily life, in sports and recreational activities, and what participation the interested party presents in recreational and daily life activities when using the groin or hip area. It has been demonstrated that this scale has qualities of validity, reliability, and responsiveness [34].

4. Rehabilitation of total hip arthroplasty

Once the hip joint degeneration becomes very disabling for the patient and when the medical treatment is no longer able to eliminate the pain or satisfy the functional needs, the situation becomes intolerable for the patient, and he/she decides to undergo surgery.

At present, surgery offers a solution to the problem due to technological advances, new materials, designs, and surgical techniques with excellent results. The hip arthroplasty aims to achieve a mobile and painless neoarticulation, with sufficient muscle function to perform daily activities in a satisfactory manner. However, the operation does not restore flexibility, strength, endurance, or normal gait pattern for daily life, in addition to the fact that each of the surgical access routes has advantages and disadvantages and often causes additional injuries to the soft tissue and bone, which require a healing/consolidation time during which rehabilitation plays a major role.

Rehabilitation protocols in hip arthroplasty are closely related to the history of the hip, the surgical techniques, the pre- and postoperative manifestations, and above all, the results. In this sense, there is not the same protocol for a hip surgery for primary coxarthrosis, a hip dysplasia, a revision or a medial fracture. That is why we say that we do not rehabilitate a hip prosthesis but a patient with a hip prosthesis, because although the surgery restores the anatomical characteristics, the recovery of function is part of the rehabilitation process. O'Halloran [35] divides the operated patients into three levels:

- Level 1: They are the youngest, active, without comorbidities, fast follow-up (< one night), and who go to the outpatient clinic once authorized.

- Level 2: Those who need more follow-up, with comorbidities and risk of clot formation, and who go to outpatient of forming clots, and who normally require home care.

- Level 3: Older adult patients, who need closer monitoring, often with more comorbidities, memory loss, and neurological impairment, requiring more prolonged home rehabilitation.

Colibazzi et al. [36] in 2020 raise several questions that have not yet been elucidated and with which we agree, such as: Which groups or subgroups of patients need intensive rehabilitation, which need home supervision, and which need only activity monitoring in a recovery center? What would be the most appropriate kinesthetic tools to use for these patients? (physical agents, manual therapy, therapeutic exercise, etc.). What should be the optimal duration of rehabilitation treatment in different patient populations? (young adults, elderly, elderly, with or without cognitive impairment, etc.), and what kind of recreational and/or sporting activities would the patient be able to engage in to maximize the longevity of their prosthesis?

In the past, analgesics were administered when the patient was in pain; now the drugs are administered before, during, and after surgery, which help the kinesiologist to speed up the programmed protocols.

Rehabilitation treatment in hip arthroplasty begins on the day of surgery, once the patient leaves the recovery room. The approach begins with patient education, explaining the type of surgery performed, the immediate care to be considered during the hospital stay, as well as at home, and the rehabilitation treatment to be carried out during recovery. Patient education is one of the pillars of rehabilitation, since its success will depend on the patient's understanding and respect for the prosthesis instability positions generated using the different surgical approaches. In our hospital, hip surgeons use the posterior approach that forces us to restrict certain activities for approximately 21 days, since we must wait for the healing of the affected soft parts. The patient is instructed not to flex the hip beyond 90 degrees, not to reach adduction or neutral internal rotation of the hip in this type of approach.

We divide the rehabilitation treatment into phases and/or stages, called hospitalization and/or home and functional recovery. Each of them has an estimated duration and in them we carry out the various activities scheduled in the protocol, but sometimes the deadlines and activities may be affected by the clinical evolution of the patient.

In the first meeting already in the patient's room, we control the functioning and position of the drainage, we focus on the prevention of phlebitis, which, apart from the pharmacological treatment with low-molecular-weight heparin, and we control the position in the bed, with slight elevation of the lower limbs, added to isometric contractions several times a day and the placement of compressive bandage or elastic stockings of containment.

We begin with early lower limb mobilization work to promote drainage of fluids that are extravasated by surgery through distal pumping from the foot and ankle, along with work of isometric quadriceps. We encourage the patient to perform active or active-assisted mobilization in triple flexion of the lower limb if the patient is unable to initiate mobilizations of the entire kinematic chain, and then, we stimulate abduction-adduction to the midline and finally hip extension with the bridge exercises. We then stimulate upper body and trunk work, and, in older adults, we also implement a series of respiratory exercises to maintain respiratory volumes and capacities, as well as thoracic flexibility. If the patient is in a hemodynamic condition to change position, we start sitting on the edge of the bed that same afternoon, always taking care of the unstable positions of the prosthesis, and stimulating the load on the operated limb in the short balance since the patient tries not to unload the operated limb because of the pain in the surgical area and because of all the postoperative hematoma.

The following day we repeat this sequence and progress to the standing position, which is usually done with the external support that the patient needs (walker, crutches, or canes), since in young adults the Canadian canes are the best option, and in older adults, the walker is the best option. In this standing position, we first look for stability in the operated limb with weight-bearing, anteroposterior and lateral imbalances and pre-walking exercises, and then we start walking. Once the patient is clinically stabilized and the complementary examinations are in order, the patient is discharged from the Hospital and transferred to his home to continue with the rehabilitation treatment.

At home we will first try to manage the behavior of the postoperative hematoma, insisting the patient to move according to tolerance, but that the stay in bed is only for moments, since not being able to change the supine position at night, rest becomes difficult.

Postural alterations are one of the most common complications we encounter when rehabilitating prosthesis. Depending on the type of surgery (primary, revision, reconstruction, etc.) and the time taken to make the decision to have surgery, the patient will arrive at the operation with vicious postures and soft tissue retractions, often due to the shortening of the limb because of joint destruction. Other times this sensation of having a shorter limb will be caused by the muscular tension of the pelvic muscles that insert into the femur and condition its position in space, leading to obliquity in the frontal plane, generating local and distant defense reactions (lumbar spine and knee). We started the flexibility work for the musculature that previously presented shortening due to joint degeneration and that altered the position of the pelvis in space. We emphasized stretching of the hip flexor muscles as these are the muscles that predispose to a limitation in extension, altering the gait pattern, generating a sensation of shortening once the surgery restores the femoral offset. We also address the adductors as their flexor component conditions the obliquity of the pelvis, perpetuating this deformity. The shortened abductors do not allow the pelvis to horizontalize in the frontal plane, giving the sensation of a longer limb. All these postural alterations generate different types of defects:

- Flexion contracture is the most frequent and is usually present in the preoperative period. It is often accompanied by a flexion contracture of the homolateral knee or of the contralateral hip. When these alterations do not exceed 10°, they have functional repercussions such as a Trendelenburg gait, reduction of the operated limb in the gait, not reaching neutral hip extension, compensating with a lumbar hyperlordosis. When the stiffness is more accentuated and the kinesics treatment fails to reverse the situation, tenotomies are performed to allow the hip to reach the neutral position of 0° of extension.

- The abduction contracture, less common but more difficult to resolve, is often accompanied by prosthesis with a long femoral neck that lateralizes the greater trochanter or a joint descent that elongates the gluteal fan, generating a lot of insertional pain. At first, it is tolerated to allow the resumption of walking with external support, accepting that the pelvis continues oblique, with an incurvation of the lumbar spine and with a compensation of the healthy lower limb by placing a heel supplement. Limb abduction is achieved progressively through analytical joint flexibility work. We then begin to analytically strengthen the hip abductors to achieve frontal plane stability, and the other muscles involved in the different phases of gait at the hip, knee, ankle, and foot.

- Internal rotation contracture is often accompanied by a lack of external rotation which is closely related to an inadequate position of the femoral stem, or to a deficiency of the external rotators damaged by the posterolateral approach. In the early postoperative period, this situation jeopardizes the stability of the prosthesis during gait and promotes dislocation. In addition, we control the position in bed with a separator (cushion) or we also use an anti-rotation boot, and we teach the patient that the changes of decubitus and the incorporations should be made keeping both lower limbs together with the cushion between the knees to avoid adduction and internal rotation movements. The patient should be instructed not to turn on the operated limb when walking, but on the controlled limb. As soon as possible, and according to the healing time of the surgical approach, we start with the analytical work of reactivation and strengthening of the external rotators.

Once these instructions have been fulfilled, we begin the functional recovery stage, where we focus on neuromuscular proprioceptive training, increase flexibility and general agility, and seek readaptation to daily activities as well as readaptation to recreational and sports activities. It is at this stage that we encounter the following complications:

- Static and dynamic Trendelenburg sign.

- Discrepancy of limbs.

- Inability to achieve certain activities of daily living.

- Impingement of the psoasiliac muscle.

- Muscular insufficiency.

Bhave et al. [37] suggest that 47% of the Trendelenburg exhibited by the patient post-surgery is due to Psoas shortening, and 36% is due to Gluteus medius insufficiency. The shortening/retraction of the psoas generates an alteration in the mechanics of the hip since the dynamic extension of the same is lost, and this leads to the non-activation of the gluteus medius, so that a Trendelenburg gait will persist. Furthermore, following the concepts of Janda, Vladimir [38], the crossed syndrome of MMII due to psoas retraction places the gluteus maximus in a position of elongation, reducing its biomechanical advantage. It is therefore crucial that the patient achieves hip extension to avoid compensation.

Regarding limb discrepancy, it is described that between 5% and 13% of total hip arthroplasties present a measurable leg length discrepancy. Those patients who come to surgery with general muscle weakness usually have an increase in length due to compensations in the position of the pelvis in space. If the lengthening is greater than 1 cm, it is preferable to add partial contralateral compensation. If the problem is postural, corrective stretching, analytical muscle strengthening and manual therapy are the usual kinesics approaches.

The ability to perform activities of daily living 1 month after surgery is often hindered by different factors such as soft tissue edema, postoperative pain, fear of adopting certain risky positions, and soft tissue stiffness. Manual lymphatic drainage in the early postoperative stages helps fluid drainage and pain management due to residual hematoma.

For the patient to recover hip rotations, we use different positions such as ventral decubitus, since here we have a better control of the pelvis position, and we can perform stretching maneuvers of the soft tissues and thus elongate the scar tissue generated by the initial restrictions. Another position is sitting with a significant opening of both knees to allow the patient to put on socks or shoes. This will give the patient back the necessary functionality in his daily activities and be able to be independent.

Psoas impingement is an entity that is being seen more frequently following hip arthroplasty. The involvement of the iliopsoas tendon has begun to be considered as one of the factors that trigger painful symptomatology in the hip, since it is often associated with pathologies within the joint, due to the close relationship of the cotyloid girdle with the joint capsule [39]. Mardones et al. found that 50% of intra-articular hip pathologies were related to psoas tendinopathy, in addition to the fact that the tendon of the *muscle*, in many cases by itself, could injure the cotyloid buckle [39]. Another work by Chalmers & cols. found up to 4.4% of patients with pain referred to the groin underlying the friction of the iliopsoas tendon with the acetabular component in joint replacements, often triggering tendon injuries. The pain was classically located in the groin when climbing stairs and when the patient attempted to use a vehicle by getting in or out of it. Resisted hip flexion, especially in long lever (terminal extension of the knee elevating the entire limb), and elongation of the iliopsoas tendon in supine when performing hip extension confirm the painful symptoms [40]. Therefore, these authors found a 50% improvement in terms of pain and joint function by means of a physiotherapy program added to NSAIDs and injection in the iliopsoas tendon sheath, with a medium-term follow-up [40]. Tendonitis or impingement may result from a prominent or malpositioned acetabular component, retained cement, an acetabular cage, a prominent femoral component collar, an oversized acetabular component, or a femoral head which is larger than the native head [41].

Phillippon et al. described a progressive protocol to strengthen the gluteus medius muscle, which identified that minimizing the concurrency of the iliopsoas muscle reduces the risk of developing or aggravating hip flexor tendinitis [42]. In their experiment in healthy individuals, they sought to isolate the work of the gluteus medius muscle through a series of rehabilitation exercises [42]. It was found that hip flexion in the supine position, lateral decubitus abduction with hip external rotation, and clam exercises (lateral abduction with approximately 45 degrees of hip flexion with knees at 90 degrees), exercises used to work the hip abductors, also activate the iliopsoas muscle to a greater or lesser extent, which is why the authors of the study suggest not performing them in patients with hip flexor involvement. They suggest that the exercise protocol should be progressive, seeking activation from low to high intensity, such as starting with terminal knee extension exercises with progressive load, then moving on to resisting hip flexion, and then working on internal/external hip rotations, clam exercises with the hip in neutral position, hip bridges in supine with both lower limbs, and then initiate hip extension with resistance, hip abduction against gravity combined with slight extension, hip abduction in lateral decubitus but adding internal rotation, and hip bridges with the request of only one limb [42].

Muscle insufficiency is a very common problem in patients who have undergone hip arthroplasty. This physical quality can be affected by numerous factors such as age, physical and nutritional condition, pain, joint stiffness, disuse due to immobilization, decrease in body mass index, and shortening of the limb due to joint degeneration leading to mechanical muscle insufficiency. If these alterations are not corrected, they can lead to complications such as mechanical loosening of the prosthesis and promote joint instability. Although there is still no consensus among orthopedic surgeons as to whether patients should be rehabilitated or not, and if so, at what stage of this intervention physiotherapy should be indicated (preoperative stage, immediate postoperative stage, and rehabilitation in specialized centers), there is evidence that therapeutic exercise, guided by kinesiologists, accelerates the recovery of patients by reincorporating them into their daily activities compared to patients who are only instructed to walk.

Assessing hip function 1 year after surgery is a good outcome measure [43]. Studies were carried out comparing the effectiveness of a home rehabilitation program with an early therapeutic exercise protocol during hospital stay, measuring variables such as muscle strength, cadence, and walking speed, in patients who underwent hip arthroplasty. *Unlu et al. in their work evaluated* 26 patients who underwent the *intervention* between 1 and 2 years prior to the study. They were divided into three groups: one with a home exercise program, the other was assigned a kinesiologist at the hospital where they were hospitalized, and the remaining group was the control group, without approaching them. After evaluating them 6 weeks after starting the work, they concluded that both the therapeutic exercise group and the group that was controlled by the kinesiologist in the hospitalization had the best results, confirming what was stated in the hypothesis of the work [43].

The group of Jan and collaborators suggest to patients who undergo hip arthroplasty surgery that they should continue with a series of active muscle strengthening exercises that should be maintained over time [44]. The protocol is based on a series of rehabilitation exercises for the patient to perform at home, basically emphasizing the muscles that stabilize the pelvis in space, basically in the frontal plane, including gait as the main factor to be improved. With this, they suggest that muscle strength levels are improved, increasing the functional capacity of the intervened patients. They suggest that the stimuli of three times a week should be respected *to* show good results [44].

Our Kinesiology Unit works as a team with the Orthopedic and Traumatology Service of the Hospital, intervening in this surgery from the immediate postoperative period and in the immediate postoperative period, in which case they attend for rehabilitation at our center until they are discharged both from rehabilitation and from the surgeon. This is why we maintain that personalized rehabilitation is one of the pillars of success in this intervention, as patient education, motivation, and compliance with work protocols reduce the risks associated with muscular insufficiency.

Just as hip arthroplasty achieves immediate pain relief and generates immediate recovery of hip function allowing the patient to return to daily activities without inconvenience, the surgery compromises various musculotendinous structures, full of mechanoreceptors, which leave patients vulnerable because proprioception is affected. These alterations generate abnormal proprioceptive signals that not only affect sensory function, but also motor control, as sensory information is essential for movement programming.

We know from several studies that currently both hip and knee joint replacements are procedures with a high success rate [45]. Substantial improvements have been observed in pain tolerance, improvements in joint function, correction of axes, and early return to a social life of relationship, without ignoring that each case is particular and that subjects can be found that after 1 year of the intervention discomfort is still present [45]. *Despite* the good results mentioned above, a percentage of post-intervention falls have been observed, although smaller. Cases of falls in the hospitalized patients of 1% in hip arthroplasty and 3% in knee arthroplasty were reported. After discharge, these falls are comparable to those patients with severe hip or knee osteoarthritis. Lo et al. found that 40% of patients operated on for hip arthroplasty, 50% of patients, who had fallen before hip surgery, and 20% of those symptomatic patients, who had not yet undergone hip surgery, fell within the first year after surgery [45].

It is well known that alterations in proprioception lead to alterations in coordination and balance, as well as being one of the reasons why patients, within a year of surgery, suffer some kind of fall, with all the consequences that this entails. Labanca et al. suggest that when patients undergo surgery for the placement of a joint prosthesis, not only the osteoarticular and neuromuscular components are compromised, but also proprioception is altered, since in the different surgical approaches the receptors responsible for the control and regulation of the movement system are affected [46]. They reported that sensory and sensory afferents and efferent, which are fundamental in motor control, are lost. Among the most affected qualities are coordination and balance, which place these patients in a state of vulnerability to falls, which in many cases are life-threatening. Because control is affected by the lack of afferences, joint movements often become clumsy and uncontrolled, which affects the quality of gait and leads to the risk of falls. Alterations have been found in gait such as decreased step cadence, reduced speed, low resistance, decreased support time on a single limb while generating oscillation of the contralateral limb, and strides of low length [46]. Therefore, these authors recommend including balance rehabilitation exercises in all phases of the process, with a structured follow-up of the progression, since in their work they were unable to discern whether the sensorimotor alterations were due to the intervention itself or to the interruption of the rehabilitation treatment [46].

4.1 Outcome measures

For patients undergoing hip arthroplasty, there are a number of rating scales for the success or otherwise of the surgery. In rehabilitation, the most widely used for these patients is the Harris Hip Score (HHS), which was introduced in 1969 to assess traumatic hip pathology based on the Harris Hip Score (HHS). During 1969, traumatic hip pathology was evaluated on the basis of four dimensions of hip pathology, which were dimensions (pain, function, range of motion, pain, function, range of motion, and absence of deformity) and uses a range of scores between 0 (worst functional range of scores), between 0 (worst possible functional capacity), and 100 (best possible functional capacity) [47].

The HHS is a valid instrument that is sensitive to changes in our setting and in patients at the start of rehabilitation after hip arthroplasty, although its behavior is like the physical function and pain dimensions of the Medical Outcomes Study-Short forem-36 (MOS SF-36). The choice between instruments, among which the Western Ontario and McMaster University (WOMAC) cannot be forgotten, may depend above all on contextual factors (Navarro Collado & cols.).

Probably, if a global view of the patient's quality of life is of interest, the MOS SF-36 is the instrument of choice, while the WOMAC would offer greater sensitivity to changes. The HHS, if it is conducted externally by professionals, may be of interest when we want to minimize some biases in patients' responses, such as socially desirable responses, and when we want to make comparisons [47].

4.1.1 Return to sport after RTC

The increasing indications for this procedure, the advancement in surgical techniques, increasingly sophisticated and durable designs and materials, and the high rate of proven success nowadays lead patients to attempt to return to recreational and/or sporting activities as soon as possible if their general physical condition permits and is a topic of debate between patients and orthopedic surgeons. There are several articles in the literature regarding recommended athletic activities for patients undergoing hip replacement surgery. One such study in 2001 was conducted by reviewing the scientific literature and conducting a survey of members of the Hip Society, the Knee Society, and the American Society of Shoulder and Elbow Surgeons [48]. Based on these surveys, the authors then provided recommendations for athletic activities for these patients.

These authors revealed that in 1999 the Hip Society surveyed 54 members regarding their recommendations for athletics and sports participation for patients who had hip replacement surgery. They divided the activities into four categories: permitted, permitted with experience, not recommended, and inconclusive. Due to relatively a small number of responses, no definitive statistical conclusion could be drawn. Clifford and Mallon and cols. [49] in 2005 provided guidance for sport participation after THR, based on a review of the literature and their own experiences. These recommendations did not vary significantly from the findings of Healy et al. [48].

In 2007, the Hip Society and the American Association of Hip and Knee Surgeons conducted a consensus-based survey of orthopedic surgeons and presented the Journal of Arthroplasty on return to athletic activity. The respondents concluded that there were no prospective randomized studies at that time that outlined guidelines for safe and appropriate activities for patients undergoing total hip arthroplasty. Recommendations at that time were based on personal preferences and surveys of surgeons' beliefs [50].

According to Vu-Han and cols. [51] in their 2020 paper they state that most surgeons surveyed in their study (81.9%) were in favors of return to sporting activity after arthroplasty. They consider the risks associated with sporting activity after THR to be minimal (1%), with periprosthetic fractures being the most important complications, followed by prosthetic dislocation and polyethylene wear. Some surgical decisions regarding implant fixation, stem type, femoral head diameter, and bearing surface tribology were influenced by expectations of return to sporting activity. What these authors observed is that there is increasingly liberal advice for the practice of high-impact sports. In our unit, we used the Consensus of the American Society for Hip Surgery where we base our classification on the traffic light giving each activity the corresponding color for when the patient can return to physical activity. We classified them as permitted (green) such as golf and swimming, recommending with experience (yellow) like weightlifting a not permitted (red) for contact sports.

5. Conclusion(s)

Rehabilitative management of the various hip pathologies is still evolving, and we are aware that more research is needed to achieve better results in our patients. We believe that there is an association between the pathological alterations we observe in FAI, hip stabilizer muscle dysfunction, and micro-instability. We kinesiologists have become expert rehabilitators of hip arthroplasty, developing increasingly intensive functional recovery protocols for these patients, but we still owe a debt, which is to prevent joint degeneration from occurring, as in this way we will always be behind the pathology and what we must achieve is to get ahead of the facts. We cannot be mere observers of the evolution of this pathology, and we must act through prevention programs, with increasingly specific protocols, and using technology as a tool, not only for evaluation but also for treatment and monitoring of the results.

Author details

Rodrigo Hamada* and Gustavo Enrique Barros
Hospital Ángel Cruz Padilla, Unidad de Kinesiología, San Miguel de Tucumán, Argentina

Address all correspondence to: rohamada@fm.unt.edu.ar

References

[1] Weir A, Brukner P, Delahunt E, Ekstrand J, Griffin D, Khan KM, et al. Doha agreement meeting on terminology and definitions in groin pain in athletes. British Journal of Sports Medicine. 2015;**49**(12):768-774. Available from: https://bjsm.bmj.com/lookup/doi/10.1136/bjsports-2015-094869

[2] Matsumoto K, Ganz R, Khanduja V. The history of femoroacetabular impingement. Bone & Joint Research. 2020;**9**(9):572-577. Available from: https://online.boneandjoint.org.uk/doi/10.1302/2046-3758.99.BJR-2020-0003

[3] Philippon MJ, Faucet SC, Briggs KK. Arthroscopic hip labral repair. Arthroscopy Techniques. 2013;**2**(2):e73-e76. Available from: https://linkinghub.elsevier.com/retrieve/pii/S221262871200059X

[4] Ryan J, DeBurca N, Mc CK. Risk factors for groin/hip injuries in field-based sports: A systematic review. British Journal of Sports Medicine. 2014;**48**(14):1089-1096. Available from: https://bjsm.bmj.com/lookup/doi/10.1136/bjsports-2013-092263

[5] Lewis CL, Sahrmann SA. Acetabular labral tear. Update. Physical Therapy. 2006;**86**(1):110-121. Available from: https://academic.oup.com/ptj/article/86/1/110/3852530

[6] Neuman DA. Kinesiology of the Musculskeletal System: Foundations for Rehabilitation. 3rd ed. Chapter 12. Elseiver, Inc; 2017. pp. 479-537

[7] Bolia J, Chahla J, Renato L, Briggs K, Phillipon M. Microinstabiity of the hip: A previously unrecognized pathology. Muscles, Ligaments and Tendons Journal. 2016;**6**(3):354-360

[8] Retchford TH, Crossley KM, Grimaldi A, Kemp JL, Cowan SM. Can local muscles augment stability in the hip? A narrative literature review. Journal of Musculoskeletal & Neuronal Interactions. 2013;**13**(1):1-12

[9] Casartelli NC, Maffiuletti NA, Item-Glatthorn JF, Staehli S, Bizzini M, Impellizzeri FM, et al. Hip muscle weakness in patients with symptomatic femoroacetabular impingement. Osteoarthritis and Cartilage. 2011;**19**(7):816-821. Available from: https://linkinghub.elsevier.com/retrieve/pii/S1063458411001099

[10] Ward WT, Fleisch ID, Ganz R. Anatomy of the iliocapsularis muscle: Relevance to surgery of the hip. Clinical Orthopaedics and Related Research. 2000;**374**:278-285. Available from: http://journals.lww.com/00003086-200005000-00025

[11] Neumann DA. Kinesiology of the hip: A focus on muscular actions. Journal of Orthopaedic & Sports Physical Therapy. 2010;**40**(2):82-114 www.jospt.org

[12] Tsai SJ, Wang CT, Jiang CC. The effect of posterior capsule repair upon post-operative hip dislocation following primary total hip arthroplasty. BMC Musculoskeletal Disorders. 2008;**9**:29, 1-6 pp. DOI: 10.1186/1471-2474-9-29

[13] Khan RJK, Yao F, Li M, Nivbrant B, Wood D. Capsular-enhanced repair of the short external rotators after total hip arthroplasty. The Journal of Arthroplasty. 2007;**22**(6):840-843. Available from: https://linkinghub.elsevier.com/retrieve/pii/S0883540306006395

[14] Pfirrmann CWA, Chung CB, Theumann NH, Trudell DJ, Resnick D.

Greater trochanter of the hip: Attachment of the abductor mechanism and a complex of three Bursae—MR imaging and MR bursography in cadavers and MR imaging in asymptomatic volunteers. Radiology. 2001;**221**(2):469-477. Available from: http://pubs.rsna.org/doi/10.1148/radiol.2211001634

[15] Kumagai M, Shiba N, Higuchi F, Nishimura H, Inoue A. Functional evaluation of hip abductor muscles with use of magnetic resonance imaging. Journal of Orthopaedic Research. 1997;**15**(6):888-893. Available from: https://onlinelibrary.wiley.com/doi/10.1002/jor.1100150615

[16] Hasselman CT, Best TM, Hughes C, Martinez S, Garrett WE. An explanation for various rectus femoris strain injuries using previously undescribed muscle architecture. The American Journal of Sports Medicine. 1995;**23**(4):493-499. Available from: https://journals.sagepub.com/doi/10.1177/036354659502300421

[17] Domb BG, Brooks A, Guanche C. Hip and pelvis injuries in sports medicine, chapter 4. In: Guanche CA, editor. Physical Examnination of the Hip. Lippincott Williams & Wilkins; 2010. pp. 62-70

[18] Whittle MW. Pathological and other abnormal gaits, chapter 3. In: Gait Analysis an Introduction. 4th ed. Elseiver; 2007. p. 101136

[19] Hoppe DJ, Truntzer JN, Shapiro LM, Abrams GD, Safran MR. Diagnostic accuracy of 3 physical examination tests in the assessment of hip microinstability. Orthopaedic Journal of Sports Medicine. 2017;**5**(11):2325967117740121. Available from: https://journals.sagepub.com/doi/10.1177/2325967117740121

[20] Riemann BL, Lephart SM. The sensorimotor system, part I: The physiologic basis of functional joint stability. Journal of Athletic Training. 2002;**37**(1):71-79. Available from: www.journalofathletictraining.org

[21] Riemann BL, Lephart SM. The sensorimotor system, part II: The role of proprioception in motor control and functional joint stability. Journal of Athletic Training. 2002;**37**(1):80-84. Available from: www.journalofathletictraining.org

[22] Saccomanni B. A review of knee proprioception before and after ACL (anterior cruciate ligament) surgery. Orthopaedic Surgery. 2019;**4**:264. Available from: http://clinicsinsurgery.com

[23] Casartelli NC, Bizzini M, Maffiuletti NA, Sutter R, Pfirrmann CW, Leunig M, et al. Exercise therapy for the management of femoroacetabular impingement syndrome: Preliminary results of clinical responsiveness. Arthritis Care & Research. 2019;**71**(8):1074-1083. Available from: https://acrjournals.onlinelibrary.wiley.com/doi/10.1002/acr.23728

[24] Kuhns BD, Weber AE, Batko B, Nho SJ, Stegemann C. A four-phase physical therapy regimen for returning athletes to sport following hip arthroscopy for femoroacetabular impingement with routine capsular closure the international journal of sports. Physical Therapy. 2017;**12**(4):683-696

[25] Cameron M. Physical Agents in Rehabilitation an Evidence-Based Approach to Practice. 6th ed. Chapter 8. 2021. Elseiver. eBook ISBN: 9780323829281

[26] Kaltenborn FM. Manual joint mobilisation of the limb joints, chapter 13. In: Examination and Manual Joint

Mobilisation in Basic Kinesic Training. 1st ed. Olso, Noruega: Olaf Norlis Bokhandel; 1986. pp. 165-172

[27] Mulligan B. Textbook of techniques, hip region chapter 11. In: The Mulligan Concept of Manual Therapy. 2nd ed. Australia: Elsevier; 2020. pp. 277-302

[28] Ylinen J. Stretching Therapy for Sport and Manual Therapies. 1st ed. Section 1. Churchill Livingstone Elsevier; 2008. pp. 3-90

[29] Lee D. The Pelvic Girdle. 3rd ed. Chapter 10. Churchill Livingstone Elsevier; 2004. pp. 163-248

[30] Boyle M. New Functional Training for Sports. 2nd ed. Chapters 6, 7. Human Kinetics; 2016. pp. 97-126. 127-162

[31] Travell JG, Simons D. Myofascial Pain and Dysfunction the Trigger Point Manual Lower Extremities, Vol. 2. 1st ed. Chapter 3. Lippincott Williams & Wilkins; 1986. pp. 28-217

[32] Fahey TD. Weight Training Basics: A Complete Program for Men and Women. 1st ed. Chapter 10. McGraw-Hill; 2005. pp. 113-124

[33] Brown LE, Ferrigno VA. Training for Speed, Agility, and Quickness. 2nd ed. Chapter 6. Human Kinetics; 2005. pp. 223-235

[34] Thorborg K, Holmich P, Christensen R, Petersen J, Roos EM. The copenhagen hip and groin outcome score (HAGOS): Development and validation according to COSMIN checklist. British Journal of Sports Medicine. 2001;**45**:478-491. DOI: 10.1136/bjms.2010.080937

[35] O'Halloran J. Current Concept in Joint Replacement. Medbridge; 2018. Available from: www.medbridgeeducation.com

[36] Colibazzi V, Coladonato A, Zanazzo M, Romanini E. Evidence based rehabilitation after hip arthroplasty. Hip International. 2020;**30**(2_suppl):20-29. Available from: https://journals.sagepub.com/doi/10.1177/1120700020971314

[37] Bhave A, Mont M, Tennis S, Nickey M, Starr R, Etienne G. Functional problems and treatment solutions after total hip and knee joint arthroplasty. The Journal of Bone and Joint Surgery, Incorporated. 2005;**87A**(2):21

[38] Page P, Frank Lardner CR. Assessment and Treatment of Muscle Imbalance the Janda Approach. Chapter 4. Human Kinetics; 2010. pp. 43-58

[39] Mardones R, Via AG, Tomic A, Rodriguez C, Salineros M, Somarriva M. Arthroscopic release of iliopsoas tendon in patients with femoro-acetabular impingement: Clinical results at mid-term follow-up. Muscles, Ligaments and Tendons Journal. 2026;**6**(3):378-383

[40] Chalmers BP, Sculco PK, Sierra RJ, Trousdale RT, Berry DJ. Iliopsoas impingement after primary total hip arthroplasty: Operative and nonoperative treatment outcomes. The Journal of Bone and Joint Surgery. 2017;**99**(7):557-564. Available from: https://journals.lww.com/00004623-201704050-00003

[41] Henderson RA, Lachiewicz PF. Groin pain after replacement of the hip: Aetiology, evaluation and treatment. The Journal of Bone and Joint Surgery British. 2012;**94-B**(2):145-151. Available from: https://online.boneandjoint.org.uk/doi/10.1302/0301-620X.94B2.27736

[42] Philippon MJ, Decker MJ, Giphart JE, Torry MR, Wahoff MS, Laprade RF. Rehabilitation exercise progression for the gluteus medius muscle with consideration for iliopsoas tendinitis: An in vivo electromyography study. The

American Journal of Sports Medicine. 2011;**39**(8):1777-1786. Available from: https://journals.sagepub.com/doi/10.1177/0363546511406848

[43] Unlu E, Eksioglu E, Aydog E, Aydoo TS, Atay G. The effect of excercise on hip muscle strength, gait speed and cadence in patient with total hip arthroplasty: A randomized controlled study. Clinical Rehabilitation. 2007;**21**:706. Available from: https://journals.sagepub.com/doi/10.1177/0269215507077302

[44] Jan MH, Hung JY, Lin JCH, Wang SF, Liu TK, Tang PF. Effects of a home program on strength, walking speed, and function after total hip replacement. Archives of Physical Medicine and Rehabilitation. 2004;**85**(12):1943-1951. Available from: https://linkinghub.elsevier.com/retrieve/pii/S0003999304003065

[45] Lo CWT, Tsang WWN, Yan CH, Lord SR, Hill KD, Wong AYL. Risk factors for falls in patients with total hip arthroplasty and total knee arthroplasty: A systematic review and meta-analysis. Osteoarthritis and Cartilage. 2019;**27**(7):979-993. Available from: https://linkinghub.elsevier.com/retrieve/pii/S1063458419309288

[46] Labanca L, Ciardulli F, Bonsanto F, Sommella N, Di Martino A, Benedetti MG. Balance and proprioception impairment, assessment tools, and rehabilitation training in patients with total hip arthroplasty: A systematic review. BMC Musculoskeletal Disorders. 2021;**22**(1):1055. Available from: https://bmcmusculoskeletdisord.biomedcentral.com/articles/10.1186/s12891-021-04919-w

[47] Navarro Collado MJ, Peiro Moreno S, Ruiz Jareño L, Paya Rubio A, Hervas Juan MT, Lopez Mateu P. Validity of the Harris hip scale in rehabilitation after hip arthroplasty after hip arthroplasty. Rehabilitation (Madrid). 2005;**39**(4):147-154

[48] Healy WL, Iorio R, Lemos MJ. Athletic activity after joint replacement. American Journal of Sports Medicine [Internet]. 2001;**29**(3):377-388. Available from: https://journals.sagepub.com/doi/10.1177/03635465010290032301

[49] Clifford PE, Mallon WJ. Sports after total joint replacement. Clinics in Sports Medicine. 2005;**24**(1):175-186. Available from: https://linkinghub.elsevier.com/retrieve/pii/S0278591904000973

[50] Klein GR, Levine BR, Hozack WJ, Strauss EJ, D'Antonio JA, Macaulay W, et al. Return to athletic activity after total hip arthroplasty. The Journal of Arthroplasty. 2007;**22**(2):171-175. Available from: https://linkinghub.elsevier.com/retrieve/pii/S0883540306006358

[51] Vu-Han T, Hardt S, Ascherl R, Gwinner C, Perka C. Recommendations for return to sports after total hip arthroplasty are becoming less restrictive as implants improve. Archives of Orthopaedic and Trauma Surgery [Internet]. 2021;**141**(3):497-507. Available from: http://link.springer.com/10.1007/s00402-020-03691-1 [Accessed: February 4, 2025]